More Praise f
How to Live Well with Chror

"There's a difference between pain and suffering. For some, pain is almost constant, but how it affects us—how we respond to it—makes all the difference. Toni shows us that difference, and she shows us what it can mean for how we live: that our lives can still be joyful."
—David R. Loy, author of *A New Buddhist Path*

"This book is an inside report from the often invisible community around us who suffer from chronic illness and pain. It is deeply human, refreshingly candid, and uncommonly wise."
—Christopher Germer, PhD, clinical instructor, Harvard Medical School

"The overarching message for those with chronic illness— and for all the rest of us as well—is that self-compassion is the most reliable refuge. Toni has been chronically ill for a long time, but her illness has not affected her perfect pitch."
—Sylvia Boorstein, *Happiness Is an Inside Job*

"The words between these covers will relieve so much pain in the world."
—Therese J. Borchard, author of *Beyond Blue*

"Through Toni's words you will find a wise friend to turn to during both the rough and the smoother times."
—Deb Shapiro, author of *Your Body Speaks Your Mind*

"Everyone with chronic illness, and those who love them, should have this book on their shelf to refer to over and over."
—Dorothy Wall, author of *Encounters with the Invisible*

"No other author I know has written as accurately and insightfully about living with chronic illness as Toni Bernhard."
—Alex Lickerman, MD, author of *The Undefeated Mind*

"As a psychotherapist, I wish this book had been written years ago. This is an invaluable guide for anyone touched by these challenges."
—Arnie Kozak, author of *Mindfulness A to Z*

"If you or someone close to you is coping with chronic difficulties, this book is not to be missed."
—Phillip Moffitt, author of *Emotional Chaos to Clarity*

"Toni Bernhard shows how limitation can open onto limitlessness—
how suffering can open onto well-being."
—Thomas Bien, author of *Mindful Therapy*

"If you have chronic illness, this is the book to
keep within arm's reach at all times."
—Danea Horn, author of *Chronic Resilience*

"This excellent guidebook is an absolute must-read
for every person facing these difficult circumstances."
—James Baraz, author of *Awakening Joy*

"Toni Bernhard shares her own powerful experience of how
mindfulness practice can deeply support anyone with chronic illness."
—Sharon Salzberg, author of *Real Happiness*

"Warm, stunningly comprehensive, wise, and practical."
—Carlin Flora, author of *Friendfluence*

"Practical and inspiring teachings both for those who have chronic
illness and for everyone who suffers and struggles in their lives."
—Mary Grace Orr, teacher at Spirit Rock Meditation Center

"Written with generosity of spirit and mind, *How to Live Well* offers
life-saving, soul-nourishing, helpful help. Each chapter provides practical
techniques not only for surviving chronic illness, but for becoming a more
compassionate person along the way. This book is a true gift."
—Joslyne Decker, author of *Fight Like a Mother:*
How to Be a Mom with a Chronic Illness

"Whether you're navigating challenges with your partner, physician,
or friends, dealing with rampant emotions, or simply learning to
accept and value the life that you have, this is the book for you."
—Joy Selak, author of *You Don't LOOK Sick*

"Chock-full of practical wisdom that will bring light and
direction to anyone lost in the darkness of chronic pain and illness."
—Susan Bauer-Wu, author of *Leaves Falling Gently*

"Toni Bernhard speaks honestly and humbly, leading to a wonderfully
balanced series of suggestions presented with compassion and a deep
understanding of the complexities of living well while sick. I will recommend
this book to friends, family members, students,therapists, and clients."
—Lizabeth Roemer, author of *The Mindful Way through Anxiety*

How to Live Well with Chronic Pain and Illness

How to Live Well
with
Chronic Pain and Illness

A MINDFUL GUIDE

Toni Bernhard

Wisdom Publications
199 Elm Street
Somerville, MA 02144 USA
wisdompubs.org

Library of Congress Cataloging-in-Publication Data
Bernhard, Toni.
  How to live well with chronic pain and illness : a mindful guide / Toni Bernhard.
    pages cm
  ISBN 1-61429-248-5 (pbk. : alk. paper)
  1. Chronic diseases—Social aspects. 2. Chronic diseases—Psychological aspects. 3. Chronically ill—Care. I. Title.
  RA644.5.B48 2015
  616'.044—dc23

                            2015006367

ISBN 978-1-61429-248-7   ebook ISBN 978-1-61429-263-0

19 18 17 16 15   **33614056425464**
 5 4 3 2 1

Cover design by Phil Pascuzzo. Interior design by Gopa&Ted2, Inc.
Set in Sabon LT Pro 10.8/16.

For my children Jamal and Mara...

Generous
Kind-hearted
Honest
Dependable.
You can count on me.
I can count on you.
You have made this a good life indeed.

Table of Contents

xi

INTRODUCTION

Making Peace with a Life Upside Down

But do not ask me where I am going
As I travel in this limitless world
Where every step I take is my home.
—ZEN MASTER DOGEN

YOU'RE NOT SUPPOSED to fall ill on a trip to Paris. You're supposed to fall in love—if not with that special someone, then with the city itself. Unfortunately, I fell ill. This was in May of 2001, and I'm still sick. A seemingly harmless viral infection compromised my immune system and turned into a chronic illness that keeps me mostly housebound and often bedbound. It felt as if my life had been turned upside down. I was supposed to be in the classroom; instead, I was in the bedroom. I was supposed to be active in my community; instead, I rarely left the house. I was supposed to be spending time with my newborn grandchild; instead, I rarely saw her.

Many people think it's somehow their fault when they become chronically ill. They see it as a personal failing on their part. We live in a culture that reinforces this view by bombarding us with messages about how, if we'd just eat this food or engage in that exercise, we need never worry about our health. For many years, I thought that the skillful response to my illness was to mount a militant battle against it. All I got for my efforts was intense mental suffering—on top of the physical suffering I was already experiencing.

The pivotal moment for me came when I realized that, although I couldn't force my body to get better, I could heal my mind. From that moment, I began the process of learning (to reference the title of my first book) "how to be sick," by which I mean how to develop skills for living gracefully and purposefully despite the limitations imposed by chronic illness. (Please note: I'll be using the terms *chronic illness* and *chronically ill* throughout the book; both terms include *chronic pain*.)

None of us can escape disappointment and sorrow in life. They come with the territory. They're part of the human condition, largely because we don't control a good portion of what happens to us. If there's no escaping our measure of disappointment and sorrow, then the path to peace and well-being must lie in learning to open our hearts and minds to embrace whatever life is serving up at the moment. This is a mindfulness practice—mindfulness infused with compassion for ourselves.

Opening in this way is not easy, and I don't always succeed. And yet when I'm able to be fully present for my experience, even if it's unpleasant and even if it's not what I'd hoped for, I feel at home in the world. I vividly remember the first moment when I accepted my life as it is—chronic illness included. I felt a huge burden lift. For the first time since I became sick, the conviction that I absolutely needed to recover my health in order to ever be happy again was absent.

In the space created by that absence, I began writing about chronic illness. I write for those who are struggling with their health, for those who take care of them, and for those who wish to understand what life is like for the chronically ill. In a nutshell, it can feel as if all our cherished plans have been upended, leaving us with a life that is at once confusing and chaotic. For this reason, I refer to chronic illness as "a life upside down."

Mindfulness is the key to developing skills for living a rich and fulfilling life in the midst of this upheaval. Mindfulness doesn't just refer to being aware of what's going on around us and in our bodies; it includes paying attention to what's going on in our minds. When we become aware of the mental and emotional challenges that accompany chronic illness, not only is it easier to adjust to and accept our new lives, but we're much more likely to make skillful decisions and wise choices along the way.

Mindfulness is usually defined as paying attention to our present-moment experience. But mindfulness is more than simply paying attention: it's paying attention *with care*. In other words, our intention matters. Are we paying attention with the intention to ease suffering in ourselves and others, or are we passive and indifferent observers of life? Without a benevolent intention, mindfulness can become a heartless practice. Are we to watch a child run into the street and—instead of yelling "Stop!"—passively note, "Child running into the street"? Of course not. This is why mindfulness means *caring attention*.

Caring attention paves the way for the sense of well-being that arises when we treat ourselves and others with kindness and compassion. Caring attention also paves the way for the arising of equanimity. No matter how frustrated and unhappy we feel at the moment, minds are flexible and can change. We can learn not to be lost in painful regrets about the lives we can no longer lead, nor to be overwhelmed with fear and worry about the future. We can move from being caught in relentless stress and anxiety about our health to a place of peace with our lives, however that life happens to be at the moment.

This book covers a broad range of topics related to chronic illness and to the chronic array of challenges that life has in store for all of us. Inspired by nearly twenty-five years of Buddhist study and practice, here is my recipe for peace of mind:

- *One dose stark reality.* Our lives, and the people in them, are uncertain, unpredictable, and do not always conform to our desires or our liking; acknowledging and accepting this is the first step toward making peace with our circumstances.
- *One dose practical skills.* Learning to pay caring attention to our lives through mindfulness practice, cultivating kindness and compassion for ourselves as well as others, and resting in the peace of mind that comes with equanimity are skills that every one of us can learn, no matter how discouraged or unhappy we are at the moment.
- *One dose humor.* Humor is good medicine for the heart and the mind.

May you find a place of peace even in the midst of your health struggles. May every step you take become your home.

I. Skills to Help with Each Day

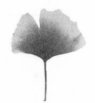

I

Educating Family and Friends about Chronic Pain and Illness

The only way to make sense out of change is to
plunge into it, move with it, and join the dance.

—ALAN WATTS

WHEN CHRONIC ILLNESS initially strikes, it feels like a crisis. Family and friends are scrambling to adjust to the many sudden and unexpected changes in your life. They may be confused about why you're not recovering. Family members, in particular, may also be frustrated over their inability to make you better and may be worried—even scared—about what the future holds.

As the months go by and the feeling of being in a crisis subsides, you may find it difficult to convey to family and friends what your day-to-day life is now like. Unless they've experienced it themselves, it's difficult for people to fathom the debilitating effects—physical and mental—of unrelenting pain and illness. Usually, the only person who truly understands is a caregiver who sees you all day long. (I've watched many a friend give me a blank look when I share that I feel as if I've had the flu, without respite, since 2001.)

I've learned that the burden is on me to make my medical condition visible to family and friends, especially because my chronic illness, as is often the case, is invisible. If I don't make the effort to educate them, their expectations of me may be way out of line with what I can handle.

In addition, educating those I'm closest to eases the emotional distress that accompanies feeling misunderstood. In the middle of Thanksgiving dinner in 2013, I had to get up from the table mid-meal because I was too sick and in too much pain to continue to sit upright. Despite this, I felt okay about leaving without explanation (which meant I didn't interrupt the ongoing conversation), because I knew that my husband, my son, and my daughter-in-law would know exactly what was going on with me. Although there were others at the table who may have thought it odd that I suddenly disappeared, knowing that these three understood gave me the courage to get up and take proper care of myself—and allowed me to do so without adding mental suffering to the physical suffering I was already experiencing.

Here are several suggestions for helping family and friends understand what your life is like. If you're reluctant to try talking with them, I recommend following Alan Watts's suggestion from the epigraph that begins this chapter: plunge into it. The changes in your life have already taken place, so you might as well do what you can to help those you love "join the dance."

Share information with them from the internet or other sources.

A good way to educate family and friends about chronic illness is to use a third-party source, such as the internet or a book. If you and a particular friend or family member have unresolved emotional issues or conflicts, using a neutral third party to convey important information keeps the focus on the issue at hand—educating the other person about your chronic illness and its effect on your life.

A quick search of the internet will yield a host of associations and organizations devoted to every conceivable medical condition. Select a few pages to print out, or forward a few links to family and friends. If you have a book that contains information you'd like them to know, buy them a copy or, alternatively, photocopy relevant pages. When you send them what you've chosen, I suggest enclosing a short note that's light in tone but also lets them know it's important to you for them to read what you're sharing. To keep it light, you could joke that "there won't be a test!"

Communicate in writing.

Many years ago, two friends of mine were in couples therapy. They were unable to talk to each other about their marital problems without one of them shouting recriminations and the other shutting down emotionally. The therapist told them that, instead of trying to speak to each other about the conflicts in their marriage, they should try to communicate by writing letters to each other. It turned out to be a major first step in healing their relationship.

If you feel at an impasse with a friend or family member, or simply feel uncomfortable talking to the person in question, consider writing a letter or sending an email. Be sure it's not accusatory. In composing it, use the word "I" more than the word "you." Describe your day-to-day life with chronic illness, explain what a difficult adjustment it's been for you, and convey how much you wish you could be as active as you once were.

You might also explain that the way you're going to feel on any given day is unpredictable, and that this means you can't be sure if you'll feel okay on a day when you've made plans to see other people, no matter how much you've rested in advance. In chapter 34 on setting the record straight, I write in detail about this particular misconception: people assume that with enough rest, we can always keep our commitments. In my experience, the hardest concept for most family and friends to comprehend is that we can spend weeks in "full rest mode" before a visit or a gathering but still be virtually nonfunctional when the day arrives.

I suggest concluding by going over what your friend or family member might expect when the two of you are together. For example, you could say that, as much as you wish you weren't limited in what you can do, you may not be able to visit for as long as you'd like. In my experience, spelling out my limitations ahead of time is helpful, not just to others, but to me, because it's much easier for me to exercise the self-control it takes to bring a visit to an end if I'm aware that the person I'm with already knows this is a very real possibility.

A final point. If you decide to communicate by email, be sure not to click "send" in haste. I recommend that you print out what you've written and review and edit it before sending it off. When I read over a hard copy of what I've drafted on the computer, I almost always find that the tone isn't quite right or that it lacks one or more subtle distinctions I was trying to convey.

Ask an ally to help you educate others.

If you find it too hard to talk to family and friends about your medical condition, think about whether there's someone in your life who truly understands what you're going through. Then ask that person to help you explain to others what life is like for you. Think long and hard before you conclude that there's no such person in your life. Your ally might be a friend or family member who's just waiting for you to enlist his or her help.

Once you've found your ally, you could ask him or her to talk with others on your behalf or to be present with you when you talk with them. Having a third party involved like this facilitates good communication; it can magically turn family and friends into careful and compassionate listeners.

If your ally is present at a gathering with you, ask him or her to be supportive if you have to leave early or go lie down. You could even ask your ally to let you know if you're "wilting," as my husband calls it when he sees that I'm pressing on even though my energy stores are depleted. It's so helpful for me to be prompted by him because going beyond my limitations causes adrenaline to kick in. This fools me into thinking I'm doing fine, but using adrenaline to get by sets me up for a bad crash later on.

Work on accepting that some people you're close to may never treat you the way you'd like.

I used to spend my limited energy going over and over my grievances about how some of the people in my life treated me. "She never asks how I'm doing." "He never acknowledges my limitations." "She's never asked me to explain my illness." Then one day I realized that the true source of my unhappiness wasn't what they were saying or not saying; it was my intense desire for them to behave the way I wanted them to. I had thought that the suffering I was experiencing was caused by them, but it wasn't. It was coming from my own mind.

The fact is, you rarely know why people behave the way they do. A friend who never shows an interest in being educated about your illness may behave that way because she assumes that if you wanted to talk about it, you'd bring it up. It's also possible that your medical condition triggers her own fears about illness and mortality, or that she's too caught up in problems of her own (medical or otherwise) to be able to take the time to educate herself about your health. Just as you can't force people to love you, you can't force people to behave the way you want them to.

When I feel let down by a friend or family member, I cultivate equanimity, mindfulness, and compassion. These three practices stem from my years of immersion in the Buddha's teachings, not as a religion, but as a practical path for finding peace with my life as it is.

I recommend that you start with equanimity. With practice, cultivating the evenness of temper that characterizes equanimity can help you feel at ease in the midst of life's inevitable ups and downs, successes and disappointments. This calm and balanced state of mind paves the way for accepting that some people will treat you the way you want and some won't.

I practice equanimity by recognizing that even though it can feel as if I'm suffering because of another person's behavior, the true source of that suffering is my own wanting mind. And even though I can still feel hurt by a friend or family member's seeming lack of understanding or interest in my health, I don't actually know what's going on in that person's mind. In the end, my sense of well-being depends on my ability to accept that other people's behavior rarely conforms to the ideal I've mocked up in my mind.

Mindfulness and self-compassion are also essential tools for making peace with family and friends whose behavior isn't as supportive as you'd wish. If you're angry, frustrated, or hurt—or any combination of painful emotions—first mindfully acknowledge that this is how you feel. Pretending that you're not feeling what you're feeling tends to intensify whatever emotions are present, so do your best to fearlessly turn your attention to what's going on in your mind at the moment. Then allow compassion to arise for any suffering you're experiencing due to the presence of painful emotions. In my view, there's never a good reason not to be as kind to yourself as you'd be to a loved one in need.

Next, reflect on how there are many possible reasons why your friend or family member is not giving you the support you'd like to have. These reasons could be related to his or her own conditioning, life history, and current concerns—and the stressful emotions that can accompany all three. It's not about you, so remind yourself that there's no reason to take it personally when someone resists your attempts to educate him or her about your health struggles.

Finally, work on wishing the best for your friend or family member. More likely than not, he or she cares deeply about you but is simply unable at this point to be present for you in the way you'd like. Understanding that others have their own "demons" can lead to compassion arising for them, even though they're letting you down. Compassion for others tends to ease your own emotional pain because it takes you out of your self-focused thinking.

As you experiment with these practices, be patient. Don't blame yourself if it's too hard at this point in your life to feel compassion for a friend or family member who is disappointing you. Instead, give yourself credit for having had the courage to plunge in and try.

My heartfelt wish is that your family and friends will be open to understanding and accepting what life is like for you, but that if they aren't, you'll be able to accept them as they are without bitterness.

2

Letting Go: A Not-To-Do List
for the Chronically Ill

Wisdom is learning what to overlook.

—WILLIAM JAMES

BEFORE I GOT sick, I depended on to-do lists. Every day I'd revise and reprioritize them. Now my life is more about what *not to do* than what *to do*. Learning what not to do and then marshalling the discipline not to do it has turned out to be a far greater challenge than making my way through those old to-do lists ever was.

It's hard to live day in and day out with "don't do this" and "don't do that" directives, especially when they often entail limiting activities that were once a source of satisfaction and joy. In addition, I can feel as if I'm letting people down if I don't follow their advice, even when I feel certain that what they're telling me to do belongs on the not-to-do side of the ledger. However, long experience has taught me that all of us fare better mentally and physically when we're able to muster the courage and discipline to pay careful and caring attention to what not to do.

Do not spend your precious energy worrying about how others view your medical condition.

When I first got sick, I wasted a lot of time and energy worrying about what I perceived to be other people's opinions of why I hadn't recovered. I'd lie in bed and torture myself with thoughts: "What if they don't understand how sick I am?" "What if they think I'm a malingerer, just trying to get out of doing things?" "If I'm at all animated when people see me, will they assume I've recovered and then judge me negatively for not resuming my career?"

I replayed these and other stressful stories over and over in my mind. It took me several years to realize that I felt better mentally and physically when I kept my attention on what was going on right now in my life, instead of spending my time lost in fantasies about what other people might be thinking about me.

Do not treat discouraging and disheartening thoughts or emotions as permanent fixtures in your mind.

I can get discouraged at the prospect that I might feel sick every day of my life from now on. When this disheartening thought arises, it's often accompanied by the feeling that I don't have the mental strength to put up with one more seemingly endless day of symptoms.

A few years ago, my husband pointed out that these types of thoughts and emotions invariably make their appearance at night-time when I'm physically at my worst and that, come morning, life always looks a bit brighter. This had never occurred to me; every time I'd feel discouraged and disheartened, I'd been assuming this was the "new me"—here to stay. But my husband was right, and his observation changed the way I treated these mental states. Now I acknowledge their presence, but I hold them lightly by reminding myself that they're not permanent fixtures in my mind. They arise simply because I feel so sick at night.

This new perspective has been tremendously helpful because it also keeps me from allowing these distressing thoughts and emotions to mushroom into full-blown "gloom and doom" stories about my life—from deciding that everyone I love is fed up with my being ill, to telling myself I should throw out all the writing I'm working on because I'm too sick to finish it. Now I'm aware that the trigger for these stressful stories is nothing more than how sick and discouraged I feel at night and that I won't feel the same way in the morning.

You might benefit from tracking your thoughts and emotions. Are there certain times of day when you feel discouraged and disheartened? Are there other triggers in your life for distressing thoughts or emotions? Mindful awareness of your thinking patterns is instructive because, without mindfulness, when you're caught up in unpleasant thoughts or emotions, you're likely to feel as if they'll last forever. By contrast, when you're feeling good, you tend not to notice because you're just enjoying the moment. Thus you can sometimes feel as though stressful thoughts and emotions dominated your day when, in fact, you experienced a range of mental states.

Discouraging and disheartening thoughts and emotions are part of the human experience, and both are impermanent. So when they come to visit, there's no reason to worry that they'll take up permanent residence in your mind. Like all mental phenomena, they blow in and blow out—just like the weather.

Do not ignore your body's pleas to say no to an activity.

It's hard to turn down participating in activities that make us feel more like the healthy people around us. When I break this rule, I feel like a rebellious child, shouting at my parents, "Look at me! I can ride a bike with no hands!" A rebellious activity can take many forms. It could be staying up too late. It could be doing too much housework or gardening. It could be engaging in exercise that's too strenuous. It could be shopping with friends for too long at the mall. It's easy to go beyond our limits when we're chronically ill, partly because adrenaline kicks in and convinces us that we're doing fine. Unfortunately, when that adrenaline wears off, a "crash" is invariably in sight.

One of my most recent bouts with ignoring my body began innocently enough. Two friends were kind enough to coach me in learning qigong. I learned movements with intriguing names, such as "Against River Push Boat" and "Huge Dragon Enters Sea." Then came "Ancient Tree Coils Root." You are to imagine that you're a strong tree, sending roots down into the ground. Unfortunately (for me), you execute this by pointing the tips of your fingers toward the ground, putting your weight all on one leg, and then squatting down on the knee of that leg.

For the first few months, I put the "one leg" instruction on my not-to-do list. I stood on two legs and squatted down only partway. I was listening to my body. Then one day, I decided I wasn't progressing fast enough, so I picked up one leg and went all the way down on the other. My knee went "crunch" and for several months afterward I was limping and had knee pain to add to the symptoms of my illness. Why did I ignore my body? I was frustrated by my limitations, and so I rebelled.

Is it ever okay to say yes to an activity when your body is saying no? Each of us has to answer this for ourselves; for me, the answer is yes—on special occasions and with full knowledge that there may be payback. This is a difficult decision to make; I'll discuss it further in chapter 7, "Dealing with Tough Choice after Tough Choice."

Do not undertake a treatment just to please whoever is pressuring you to try it.

People have lots of advice for me regarding my health—from the reasonable to the absurd. I used to feel obligated to follow their advice just to please them. In retrospect, that's quite amazing: in order to please someone, I'd follow his or her advice even if my mind and body were telling me in no uncertain terms that it wasn't a good idea.

Both my body and my pocketbook have suffered as a result of having ignored this *not to do* directive. People can be very persuasive, especially if they claim that a treatment cured them. However, from years of hanging out on internet health sites, I've learned that for every prescription medication, every dietary supplement, and every alternative treatment (Western and Eastern), I can find people who say it worked, people who say it didn't make a difference, and people who say it made them worse.

I still experiment with new treatments and I intend to keep doing so, but I no longer try something simply to please the person who is pressuring me to try it. I do my own research and I consult with people I trust, including my primary care physician. For this reason, I'm happy to report that I did *not* follow the advice of someone who was sure I'd be cured if I'd only jump in a cold swimming pool of water every morning for six months!

Do not be angry when people in your life don't respond as you'd like.

It took a while, but I've finally learned that feeling angry toward people who don't act the way I want them to serves no constructive purpose. It doesn't make me any less sick, nor does it change the other person's behavior. A huge burden dropped away from me the day I stopped expecting everyone to treat me the way I wanted to be treated. And the day I stopped directing anger toward those people was the day I began to find a measure of peace in this unexpected turn my life has taken.

Again, this is an equanimity practice. Unlike in the previous chapter, however, instead of the emphasis being on accepting that not everyone will behave as I want them to, the emphasis is on *having that be okay with me.* Do I really need everyone to understand what it's like for me to be chronically ill? No. Do I really need everyone to step up to the plate and be as supportive as I'd like? No, I don't.

It takes courage to accept people as they are without anger or bitterness, even though they may be letting you down. I've let a few close friends slip out of my life altogether, while at the same time doing my best to wish them well. It's been a challenge at times, but it's better for me to stick with friends who actively support and accept me rather than spend my time with those who appear to be uncomfortable around me as I am now.

Do not get hooked into believing you always have to "think positively."

This is known in the counseling profession as the "tyranny of positive thinking." Are we never supposed to get frustrated or disheartened about our medical conditions? That would be holding ourselves to an impossible standard. People in excellent health get frustrated and disheartened at times about their lives, so of course those of us who are chronically ill do too. Our "unpositive thinking" moods can be particularly intense, because they're often triggered by stressful thoughts and emotions that arise because of our health problems.

I have days when I'm just plain weary of being sick. I've come to think of this "unpositive thinking" as a natural response to the relentlessness of chronic illness. I don't try to force myself into thinking positively at a moment like this. I wait the feeling out, knowing that, like all feelings, it's impermanent.

Some people even tell us that positive thinking can cure disease. Although the mind and the body are interconnected, I do not believe that visualizing that we're 100 percent healthy can cure chronic illness—although I've received dozens of emails trying to convince me otherwise.

Do not put your pre-illness life on a pedestal.

Most of us have a tendency to glorify the past. I used to have a recurring fantasy in which I'd recovered my health, and my husband and I had returned to our special hideaway on the island of Molokai—a rental cottage we'd discovered in 1995. It was in a lush, fragrant environment, surrounded by papaya trees. We were within walking distance of the island's only resort. In the evenings, we'd stroll to the bar, take our drinks outside, and listen to live music while watching the island's spectacular sunsets. We traveled to our hideaway almost every year until I got sick in 2001.

My fantasy of returning there persisted until one day I looked on the internet and found that an economic downturn and a dispute over land rights have changed life on Molokai. Many tourist businesses have closed, including the resort we loved so much, and hundreds of residents have lost their jobs. The pictures I saw of how the island looks today bore little resemblance to the island of my fantasy.

Life is in constant flux. The environment changes, relationships change, job conditions change, cultural norms change. There's no reason to assume that pleasures from the past would bring us the same enjoyment should we regain our health and be able to engage in them today. (For more on this phenomenon, see chapter 29, "Beware of 'Good Old Days Syndrome.'")

There's nothing wrong with enjoying fond memories of the past, but that's different from putting that past on a pedestal and convincing ourselves that life was perfect for us then—or even near perfect. When I find myself doing this, I consciously shift my attention to the present moment and try to get on with the day that's unfolding before me.

Do not call yourself names or otherwise speak unkindly to yourself when you break one of your not-to-do rules.

Please don't compound having broken a not-to-do rule by engaging in negative self-judgment. Most of us have been conditioned from childhood to be our own harshest critics. We hold ourselves to standards that we'd never think of imposing on others. Everyone breaks the rules once in a while. When you do, I hope you'll forgive yourself immediately.

That said, some people don't know how to forgive themselves. If this describes you, try this exercise. First, write down the self-critical thought you're directing at yourself. If you stayed out too long with friends, it might be: "I'm so stupid. I knew not to spend so much time at the mall with my friends, but I did anyway."

Second, call to mind a loved one—perhaps your own child or a best friend. Imagine that this person made one of those statements to you about him- or herself: "I'm so stupid. I knew not to spend so much time at the mall with my friends, but I did anyway." How would you respond? You'd probably say something along these lines: "Please don't be hard on yourself. You're not stupid. You're so isolated by illness that the prospect of spending as much time as possible with your friends was simply irresistible. Anyone might have done it."

Third, now say those very words to yourself. "I'm being too hard on myself. I'm not stupid. I'm so isolated by illness that the prospect of spending as much time as possible with my friends was simply irresistible. Anyone might have done it."

When you try this exercise, if your inner critic is strong, you may feel uncomfortable speaking to yourself in such a kind voice. It may even sound so strange and foreign that it feels fake—not genuine. That's okay. With this exercise, you're beginning the process of reversing conditioning that's been a lifetime in the making. "Fake it 'til you make it" works very well in this situation!

With practice, you can change your inner critic into an ally. This can give you the courage and the confidence to recommit to following your not-to-do list, so that you can take the best care of yourself as possible. Just remember not to hold yourself to a standard of abstract perfection. Self-compassion always comes first.

3

Asking for Help Can Be Your Gift to Others

No one has ever become poor by giving.

—ANNE FRANK

LIKE MANY PEOPLE, I always thought that asking for help was a sign of weakness and an imposition on others. Even after I became chronically ill and sometimes needed help badly, this attitude persisted. Then I had an experience that made me realize that asking for help can be an act of kindness toward others. Allowing them to help when you're struggling with your health makes them feel *less helpless* in the face of the new challenges in your life. It can mean a lot to someone to be able to aid a friend or family member who is struggling with his or her health.

Here's what happened that changed my outlook on asking for help. One day, my friend Dawn came to visit and showed me an exquisite handmade dress she'd just bought for her granddaughter at a local boutique. When I told her how much I loved it, she asked if I'd like to get one for my granddaughter Malia. I said, "That would be great," and before I could finish my sentence by adding, "but I'm not well enough to go shopping," she was out the door and on her way back to the boutique.

She returned shortly with the dress in two sizes for me to choose from. I picked one and wrote her a check. When she left to go home, she took the one I didn't want back to the boutique. That made three trips for her to the same store that day. I saw in her face that getting that dress for me to give to Malia was *a gift from me to Dawn*. She can't restore my health, but she can buy a dress for me to give to my granddaughter, and doing it made her feel good... and helpful.

And so I think it would be beneficial for we who are chronically ill to develop some skill at asking for help. We often need it, and most of those who care about us want to give it. I said "most" because every relationship is different. There may be people in your life who've never learned the joy of helping others. It's sad for them, and yet that's the way it is. In that case, think of other people to ask.

It takes practice to learn to ask for help. Most of us have to overcome a lifetime of conditioning in which we've been taught that only the weak need help. As a result, we cling to the notion "I can do everything myself," even though it may no longer be the case. Try following these steps:

1. Make a list of what you need help with: cooking, laundry, weeding, walking the dog, a trip to the hardware store, even just a shoulder to cry on. Your chances of success are higher if you give the person a specific task. We tend to think it should be obvious to others what kind of help we need, but family and friends aren't mind readers. Even if you're in a longstanding and close relationship, the other person doesn't necessarily know what would be helpful to you at this moment. Tell people what you need.

2. Write down the names of family and friends who might be

willing to help. A good starting point would be names of people who've already offered, even if their offers were made some time ago.

3. Match people with tasks based on their interests, strengths, time flexibility, and your comfort level with them if the task is of a more intimate nature, such as doing laundry. I read about a ten-year-old girl who earned her Girl Scout cooking badge by cooking for her housebound neighbor once a week.

4. Now comes the tough part of this new skill you're learning, so start modestly. Pick one thing from your list and contact the person you've chosen. Be direct—no passive-aggressive pleas allowed! And so instead of saying "If only I knew someone who could pick up a prescription for me," ask outright: "Can you pick up a prescription for me? I'm not well enough to go out." Remember, the more specific the request, the better. "Can you help with my laundry every other week?" is more likely to be successful than "Can you help with my laundry once in a while?" Even though your friend or family member is likely to say yes to both requests, the wording of the second one is too open-ended, meaning neither of you is likely to follow-up.

The odds are high that the person you've contacted will be happy—and maybe even relieved—that you've finally asked him or her for help. Think of your request as a gift from you: it gives this person a way to not feel helpless in the face of your health challenges. If you strike out, take a deep breath and try again. Even multi million-dollar baseball players get more than one strike!

It's ironic that we think we're imposing a burden on people when we ask them to do something for us—even though, if we did the very same thing for them, we wouldn't consider it a burden. On the contrary, it would make us feel good to know that our friend or family member feels comfortable enough around us to seek our help.

If you feel unworthy of being helped by others, bring to mind some examples from the past when people were helpful to you. Obviously, *they* didn't think you were unworthy. Use those memories as a starting point for changing your self-critical thinking. It's not a sign of weakness to ask for help. It's an act of self-compassion.

4

Developing the Confidence to Say No

To be yourself in a world that is constantly trying to make you something else is the greatest accomplishment.

—RALPH WALDO EMERSON

I'M TEACHING MYSELF when to say no. I was raised to accommodate others and to give their opinions about what I should or should not be doing more weight than my own. It took many years of chronic illness to realize that it's an act of self-compassion to mindfully examine what people are asking of me and then decide for myself if I should say yes or no.

As guidance in learning how to respond to people, I've been relying on the Buddha's teachings on skillful speech; he said that we should speak only when what we have to say is true, kind, and helpful. He was focusing on what we say to other people, but I've also been applying his three-part test to myself. Unless saying yes would be true, kind, and helpful to me, I'm working on saying no. Here's a look at the Buddha's test from this different point of view.

Would saying no as opposed to yes be true to yourself?

Ask yourself if you're about to say yes because doing so would be true to your values and beneficial to you. Or are you acquiescing due to social pressure? Or perhaps you feel relatively powerless in the presence of the other person (the latter is common in a medical setting).

I spent a good part of my younger years speaking or acting to please others, even when it wasn't true to my deepest values, and I suffered because of it. I once smiled in implied assent to a racist comment because the speaker was an influential elected official who had contributed money to my husband's political campaign. Although it happened over twenty-five years ago, I still feel self-incrimination arise as I write about it.

One benefit of mindfulness practice is that when you pay careful and caring attention to what's going on in the present moment, it forces you to slow down. This can prevent you from blurting out a knee-jerk reactive yes when saying no would be true to yourself.

I wish I'd learned the self-protective value of saying no before I became chronically ill. I could have avoided so much suffering—physical and mental. For example, after taking a semester off when I first became sick, I returned to the classroom and continued teaching part-time for another two years, even though I wasn't well enough to be in the workforce. This may well have contributed to how ill I still am today. A half hour before my class was to begin, I'd roll out of bed, put on a professional-looking outfit, brush my hair, have my husband drive me to the law school, teach my class while sitting in a chair, and return as quickly as I could to my bed.

I came up with strategies so I could interact with students without getting caught in prolonged conversations. For example, after class, I'd use an empty classroom to talk with students instead inviting them to my office. That way, I could get up and leave as soon as I'd answered their questions.

During those two years, I made sure the students didn't suffer as a result of having a teacher who was sick, but I sure did suffer. And why? Because I could not say no. I'd convinced myself that everyone around me thought I should be continuing with my career. I gave more weight to what I perceived to be their view of what was beneficial for me than I gave to my own body telling me to stop working. In this sense, I betrayed my body instead of being true to it.

I've also had to teach myself when to say no to doctors. In 2009, I tripped on a step and broke my ankle. After the ankle healed, one of my toes remained painfully swollen, so my primary care doctor sent me to a podiatrist. She gave me a cortisone shot in my toe, telling me it should fix the problem. The shot didn't help my toe; even worse, the cortisone exacerbated the symptoms of my chronic illness.

When I returned for a follow-up appointment a few weeks later, she hurriedly said that I needed a second cortisone shot. My body and mind were silently screaming no; yet, feeling powerless in her presence, I passively sat there and let her give me the shot. Looking back on that appointment, it's hard to believe that I didn't say no. But I didn't. And the result of the shot was the same: no relief for my toe and an exacerbation of my symptoms.

Had my mindfulness skills been stronger, I would have recognized that I needed to slow down the speed with which she was conducting the appointment by telling her I wanted to think about it for a few minutes. Then I'd have weighed the pros and cons with caring attentiveness, and I would have said no.

When you become aware that it might be time to say no, either to what you're doing (such as continuing to work) or to what others are asking of you, stop and ask yourself what would be true to yourself. Will your response reflect your values? Will it ease your suffering—mentally and physically—as opposed to intensifying it? Finally, ask yourself what the self-protective and self-compassionate response would be in this situation.

Would saying no as opposed to yes be kind and helpful to yourself?

In working with this test, I apply *helpful* to what I think would benefit my emotional and mental well-being. Then I apply *kindness* to my body. Often what's helpful to my mind is not kind to my body, and my goal is not to say yes unless all of the Buddha's criteria are met. This means that even if saying yes would be uplifting mentally, if it's not also kind to my body, I should be saying no.

Of course, the mind and body are interconnected, so separating them this way might seem artificial; yet for purposes of applying this test, it works well. For example, if someone invites me and my husband out for the evening, it might help me emotionally to say yes because I'd feel less isolated. But it would not be kind to my body—when I socialize in the evening, I invariably face a flare in my symptoms that leaves me bedbound the next day.

Similarly, shortly after my first book was released in 2010, I was contacted by the producer of a nationwide AM radio show. The show's host wanted to interview me about how I became chronically ill and then ask me questions about how the book might help people who are struggling with their health.

This invitation was definitely helpful to my emotional state; it gave me such a mental lift to know that this station wanted me on its show! I was excited to be able to share my story with others and to tell them about the new book. Then the producer informed me that I'd have to be on LIVE. The show originates in New York City; my segment would air from 6:30 a.m. to 7:00 a.m. Eastern Time. I live in California—on Pacific Time. This meant I'd have to be up and ready to be interviewed at 3:30 in the morning.

Because a good night's sleep is essential to my ability to function, I protect it dearly. I knew that, as beneficial as this opportunity sounded for my mental well-being, it would not be kind to my body. After much deliberation, I decided that the lack of kindness to my body outweighed how helpful it might be to my mind. And so I declined the offer. I felt sad at the time, but I've never regretted making the decision.

I used to let what I thought would help my emotional well-being trump what I thought would be kind to my body—and that may be warranted on truly special occasions. I've learned, though, that my body feeling at its best benefits me both physically and mentally. Despite this knowledge, there are times when the appeal of something like an evening of socializing, particularly because I'm so isolated, can blind me to the consequences that are sure to follow. This may not be the case for everyone but, for me, a day spent in bed feeling terribly sick almost always wipes out whatever emotional benefit I gained from the evening.

Once you begin to say no, it gets easier and easier. Think of it as a practice. That way, you won't hold yourself to too high a standard. Because I have a lifetime of conditioning to overcome, I still say yes sometimes when it would be self-protective and self-compassionate to say no. I've spent most of my life trying to please others, even when following their lead wasn't kind, helpful, and true to myself. But at last, I'm getting better at saying no and, when I do, it feels good—both in body and in mind.

5

When the "Want Monster" Whispers
in Your Ear

The greatest wealth is a poverty of desires.

—SENECA

WHEN I WAS a young girl, I wanted a horse. Almost every day, I begged my parents to get me one. Now I look back with sympathy at what my poor parents were forced to say to me over and over again: "You can't have a horse in the middle of Los Angeles! Where would you keep it? Where would you ride it?" At the time, none of their attempts to discourage me mattered. All I wanted was a horse. I truly believed that if I had one, I'd be happy for the rest of my life. Even more: I couldn't imagine being happy *unless* I could have that horse.

How many times have you smiled and shaken your head in disbelief at how positive you were that some material thing or some particular experience was absolutely necessary for your happiness? Now you look back and those desires are simply items on a list of "wants" that no longer have any hold over you.

It's easy for me to recall that young girl and laugh at her out-of-control desire for a horse, but the fact is, I can still want something so badly that it feels like a need over which I have no control. This type of desire is more than just a preference for, say, vanilla ice cream over chocolate. It can be so intense that I talk myself into believing that if I *can't* get what I want, I'll never be happy.

These days, most of those wants are related to the desire to regain my good health. Here are some of the "wants" that periodically come up for me since becoming chronically ill:

- Wanting to take my granddaughters places
- Wanting to travel again to Hawaii with my husband
- Wanting to be symptom-free for a few days

Is there something in your life that you want so badly that it feels as if your happiness depends on getting it?

My friend Sandy calls this the "Want Monster." When her two children were young, she used this phrase to help them become aware of their tendency to want anything that appeared pleasant to them, whether it was a material thing or an experience. If they were in a toy store and started madly grabbing for stuff, she'd remind them that this was the Want Monster showing up and that it need not be satisfied. If they thought they couldn't be happy unless they went to Disneyland, she'd remind them: it's just the Want Monster.

Our desire to satisfy the Want Monster can feel so intense that we can talk ourselves into believing that getting what we want is necessary to our very ability to be happy. This belief is reinforced by that ever-present cultural message—perhaps better characterized as "cultural bombardment"—telling us that the key to lasting happiness is getting what we want: a better car, a new relationship, an expensive piece of exercise equipment that will get us back our youthful bodies.

And yet the type of happiness that comes from satisfying the Want Monster is short-lived—because nothing is permanent. A car will go out of fashion or wear out. Even relationships that stand the test of time don't bring with them permanent, 'round-the-clock happiness. And bodies age, no matter how much we exercise them.

This conviction that the key to happiness is satisfying our desires sets us up for a big dose of disappointment and dissatisfaction with our lives. One reason for this is that most of our desires go unfulfilled—we simply don't get our way a lot of the time. In addition, our minds are as ever-changing as everything else in the universe, so even when we're able to fulfill a desire, it's unlikely to satisfy us for long. It soon gives way to a new desire. As Oscar Wilde famously said: "There are only two tragedies in life: one is not getting what one wants, and the other is getting it."

I often hear the Want Monster whispering in my ear: "If only you could get your health back, everything would be great for you from now on." When I reflect deeply, though, I realize that this is a delusion. If my health were restored, my life would still have its share of problems.

I'm not suggesting we become passive and give up our efforts to try and make things better for ourselves. I'm always on the lookout for new treatments—I consult with Dr. Google regularly. But I also know that I'm entering into the land of delusion when I find myself believing that getting my health back would make me forever happy.

In the end, the type of happiness that depends on satisfying the Want Monster is not the happiness I'm looking for; I know it would only be temporary. I'm looking for happiness that comes from being content with my life as it is, whether or not I'm able to take my granddaughters places, or travel to Hawaii, or even regain my health.

This happiness comes from acknowledging and accepting without aversion that, despite my best efforts and despite my hopes and dreams, sometimes things don't work out as I want them to. This happiness comes from making peace with the stark realities of life—that it's a mixture of pleasant and unpleasant experiences, easy times and hard times, getting what I want and not getting what I want. It's that way for everyone, and has always been. This happiness comes from opening my heart and mind to engage each day fully, even though I know it may be a day in which the Want Monster goes hungry.

No matter how tight a hold the Want Monster seems to have on us, the good news is that, with practice, we can free ourselves from its grip. Over 2,500 years ago, the Buddha said what neuroscientists are confirming today: the mind is malleable, and so it can change. The Buddha put it this way: "The mind is as soft and pliant as the balsam tree." Neuroscientists say that the mind is constantly rewiring and reconditioning itself. This means we can reverse those deeply ingrained habits that keep us believing in the delusion that our happiness depends on fulfilling our desires.

Mindfulness practice is the path to freeing ourselves from the Want Monster. The first task is to become aware that a Want Monster–type of desire has arisen. Then we can make a conscious decision not to let it talk us into believing that getting our way will solve all our problems. It may whisper in our ear that regaining our health is a have-to-have-it-or-be-miserable-the-rest-of-our-life desire, but we know that true happiness does not depend on satisfying that longing.

When we're able to treat the Want Monster as nothing more than mental chatter—an event in the mind, arising, hanging out for a while, and then passing away—we'll be free to fully engage with what this particular day has to offer.

6

Complaining Is a Recipe for Suffering

*If you are irritated by every rub, how will your mirror
ever be polished?*

—RUMI

FOR THE CHRONICALLY ill, there's lots to complain about: ongoing unpleasant symptoms, the loss of the ability to do things,
friends gone missing, unresponsive doctors, uncertainty about the
future. The list is long. In my experience, however, complaining is
rarely productive; it's almost always a recipe for further suffering
and dissatisfaction.

Most complaining centers around a desire to control what's
happening to us. One of life's stark realities, however, is that we
have limited control over how things are unfolding at any given
moment. We hear that Want Monster whispering in our ears, but
we can't seem to get our way. And so, instead, we complain.

Here's an exercise to remind ourselves that complaining isn't
a skillful way to respond to the circumstances of our lives. I

hope you'll join in. I'm going to start by making a sample list of complaints:

1. I don't want to be sick anymore.
2. I don't want to get old.
3. I haven't moved for twenty minutes on this [censored] freeway.
4. I'm put on hold for way too long whenever I call my doctor's office.
5. My partner is always complaining about my poor health.
6. I hate being in constant physical pain.
7. My friends should call more often to see how I'm doing.

Don't judge yourself negatively over the length of your list. That is, don't complain that your list of complaints is too long! That type of self-critical thinking can keep you from reaping the benefits of this exercise. It's nothing more than a list of your complaints. Hold it lightly.

The issue here is not whether your complaints are justified. Justified or not, they still reflect dissatisfaction, because underlying a complaint is the desire for life and the world to be different than they are.

Now go through your list and separate it into three parts: (1) those complaints involving circumstances over which you have no control; (2) those complaints involving circumstances over which you might have some control; (3) those complaints involving circumstances over which you have total control. It's highly likely that none of your complaints will fall under (3).

No Control

If this were my list (honestly, it's not—well, not all of it!), I'd say that I have no control over numbers 1, 2, 3, and 4. That's over half the items on the list. These four involve conditions in my life and in the world that aren't within my power to change. I can change my *response* to these four conditions (and that can definitely reduce my suffering), but I can't change the bare facts of these circumstances:

1. I've tried dozens of treatments; for now, there's no way around it: I'm chronically ill.
2. No amount of complaining will keep me from getting old.
3. I have no control over the flow of freeway traffic. Maybe there was an accident up ahead. Maybe there's road work in progress. Complaining about a traffic jam won't clear it up any sooner.
4. I don't control how long I'll be put on hold. It may be a very long time. I can spend that time fuming about it, or I can spend that time doing something pleasant, such as crocheting or surfing the internet.

Look over your own list and see how many of the items are out of your control entirely. Can you see that complaining about circumstances you cannot affect is pointless? And worse than pointless—harmful. Such complaining serves only to add suffering and dissatisfaction to an already unpleasant situation, making you more stressed, anxious, and unhappy.

Are there any items on your list that you can let go of, since you can't control them anyway? If yes, does letting them go bring a sense of relief? Whenever I use the phrase *let go*, I recall the words of Thai Buddhist monk Ajahn Chah:

> If you let go a little, you will have a little peace. If you let go a lot, you will have a lot of peace. If you let go completely, you will know complete peace and freedom. Your struggles with the world will have come to an end.

As inspiring as his words are, there may be times when you can't let go of a complaint. It's simply too hard. When that happens, simply *let it be* by acknowledging with compassion for yourself that the complaint is a source of suffering for you. This simple act in itself can keep you from ratcheting up the intensity of your complaining.

Partial Control

For this category, I would select numbers 5, 6, and 7, although I'm not convinced that some of them wouldn't fit better under "no control."

To address the items in this category, begin by recognizing that since you have only at best partial control over these complaints, you should consider letting them go. At the very least, try letting them be by not putting more energy into complaining about them.

5. What are the chances that complaining about my complaining partner will make him complain less?
6. Does it lessen my physical pain to hate it? On the contrary: it could intensify the pain. Stressful emotions, such as anger and hatred, often lead me to tighten muscles around points of bodily discomfort, increasing my overall pain load.
7. Is it fruitful to make myself miserable by complaining about my friends not calling more often since I don't control their behavior?

Because these three are categorized under "partial control," think about what kinds of skillful action might be effective. (I define "skillful action" as speech or action that eases stress and suffering for ourselves or others.) Start by acknowledging, without judgment, that things are as they are: a complaining partner, the presence of physical pain, friends who don't call often. This non-judgmental assessment facilitates dispassionate problem-solving.

5. Could I try some strategies with my partner that might help him complain less about my health, such as validating his

feelings? For example, I could say to him "It must be so hard on you for me to be sick all the time" or "I'm sorry if you miss going out together." Could I raise the idea of couples therapy?

6. Could I get a referral to a pain clinic, or try some of the mindfulness-based practices in this book that are specifically intended to help cope with pain? (See, for example, chapter 11.)
7. Could I pick up the phone and call my friends myself?

Total Control

I don't see anything on the list over which I could claim total control.

Complaining is a habit that clouds our ability to see that most of our complaints involve circumstances over which we have little or no control. If our peace of mind depends on controlling every aspect of our lives, that peace will always elude us. When we're not getting our way, instead of moving straight into complaining mode, we'd suffer less if we took a few conscious breaths and then used our mindfulness skills to calmly assess whether or not there's anything we can do about the situation. If there isn't, we can try to let it go—at least, we can try to not intensify our complaining, which only makes us feel worse.

When we're able to acknowledge and accept without aversion that our lives will include experiences that won't be to our liking, we'll be better able to take those unpleasant experiences in stride— or, as Rumi put it, not be "irritated by every rub." Then our tendency to complain will subside. What a sweet relief that would be!

7

Dealing with Tough Choice after Tough Choice

Start where you are. Use what you have.
Do what you can.

—ARTHUR ASHE

BEING CHRONICALLY ILL can feel like a full-time job—an exhausting one at that. We're constantly engaged in an ongoing evaluation of whether we're managing our health and our relationships with others as skillfully as possible. Then, based on those assessments, we have to choose the most beneficial course of action, even though the choice may not be a completely satisfying one. That's why what follows are not just choices but tough choices.

Do we talk openly about our health problems, or do we keep them private?

In chapter 1, I wrote about the importance of trying to educate those we're closest to so that we can receive the support and understanding we need. But what do we do about the many other people we encounter in life, such as coworkers and casual acquaintances? How do we respond when they ask us how we are?

On the one hand, if we talk openly about our health problems, some of them may turn away in aversion and avoid us from then on. Others may have the opposite reaction; they may become so concerned about us that we find ourselves in the role of temporary caregivers, having to reassure them that they shouldn't worry and that we're coping fine (even if we're not). Still others may take it upon themselves to lecture us on what they think we should or shouldn't be doing—and then be upset with us if we don't follow their advice.

On the other hand, if we treat our health issues as private— even acting "fake healthy" as I've been known to do—we risk misleading others about what we're capable of doing. In addition, hiding our symptoms can make us feel as if we're betraying ourselves by being dishonest about what our lives are like. Finally, by keeping quiet, we may be passing up a genuine opportunity to connect with another person and to receive much-needed support—both emotional and practical.

And so, when faced with the dilemma of how to respond to someone's inquiry about how we are, we have lots of choices. Quickly assessing the situation and then making an on-the-spot decision about what to share and what to keep private can be exhausting.

I can't offer a simple answer to this dilemma or to the other tough choices in this chapter. All we can do is try our best to evaluate our circumstances and our needs, and then choose the course of action that appears to be the most beneficial and compassionate for us.

Do we follow our doctor's treatment plan, or do we try alternative therapies?

After becoming chronically ill, I spent most of my time in bed, using my laptop to search the internet for cures. It took me several years to realize that anyone can create a website, set up a payment plan, and ask for my credit card number. *Anyone.* Treatments-for-sale can be packaged to sound irresistibly seductive. People spend thousands of dollars on false cures. I know, because I've done it.

On the other hand, I've also read about people who've been helped by alternative treatments, so disregarding them outright is not always the best decision. This tough choice makes up a major part of the workload for the chronically ill. What should we try? What should we not try? How much research should we do on a treatment option before deciding if we should try it or not? If we try something, how long should we give it before deciding whether it's helping or not? How should we budget for it? What should we tell our doctors about it? No way around it; this is exhausting work.

**Do we take medication to relieve disabling pain,
or do we stoically put up with it because the medication
makes us groggy and less functional?**

I've yet to meet anyone who likes the side effects of pain medication; even so, it's a tough choice: a body in unremitting pain or a mind like silly putty. Neither choice is satisfactory, but we still have to make it. Which choice we make on any given day may depend on several factors, such as what our "have to's" for the day look like and whether we'll be spending time with other people.

Related to this tough choice is the decision of how to allocate pain medication if we're only given a certain amount each month. Here's what Carol, who has chronic migraines, said about this:

> Insurance companies limit the amount of pain medication they will give us per month. The problem is that if you get fifteen to eighteen migraines per month as I do, the nine pills allowed must be doled out very carefully. So

not only do I have a migraine, I have to assess it: maybe it's not so bad that I need to medicate... but what if it gets worse? And how many pills have I already taken this month? If I take more than four by mid-month, I won't have enough to get through to the end... but if I let it get too bad, then the medication doesn't work as well and I am down and out for a couple of days.

I'm exhausted *for* Carol just reading this.

Do we ignore a new or worsening symptom, or do we have it checked out by a doctor?

It's not good for us emotionally to be overly focused on every little ache and pain in our bodies. In addition, we may be concerned that if we raise a new or worsening symptom, the doctor will think we're being oversensitive or even a hypochondriac—either of which might affect the quality of care we receive.

But consider this. I read in one of my chronic illness books about a woman who ignored a new symptom. She decided it was best to assume it was related to her chronic illness because she didn't want to bother her doctor. The new symptom turned out to be stomach cancer.

An issue that can arise with a worsening symptom is the need to decide whether it's related to our chronic illness or is a natural part of the aging process. Is that stiffness that wasn't there a few months ago related to our illness, or is it just a sign that our bodies are aging? Is the sudden need to take a nap in the afternoon an indication that our condition is worsening, or do people simply need to nap as they age?

The appearance of a new symptom or the recognition that an old one is worsening requires that we make another tough choice:

wait or act immediately. Each of us has to listen carefully to our bodies and decide for ourselves. It isn't easy, that's for sure.

Do we ask for help with anything that's difficult for us, or do we save up our requests and use them only when there's something we absolutely cannot do?

On the one hand, we don't want to overburden family and friends. In addition, we treasure what independence we still have. These concerns incline us toward going ahead and doing what we can, even though there may be some payback later.

On the other hand, if we're stingy in asking for help, friends and family might assume we're able to do much more than we're capable of: "You were able to go to the store, so you must be able to go to the beach for the day." Knowing that we might get this kind of reaction if we try to do even the smallest tasks makes us wonder if it wouldn't be better to always ask for help.

Do we spend what little energy we have doing necessary things like laundry or even showering, or do we use it to do something that's nourishing and fulfilling to us?

I remember facing this tough choice when my newborn son was napping. I'd think: "Great! Now I can do something for myself alone—a hot bath, a good book, maybe even my own nap!" Despite these appealing possibilities, invariably, I wound up doing things around the house that weren't otherwise getting done—a sink full of dishes, a load of laundry. In the end, I never used his naps for my own enjoyment or nourishment. Now I face this same tough choice again.

Do we use makeup and the like to cover up how sick we are or how much pain we're in, or do we let people see how we really feel?

I face this dilemma whenever I go out. I remember the "back and forth" that went on in my mind as I was getting dressed to go to an event at our local bookstore when my first book, *How to Be Sick*, was released. I thought, "If I put cover-up on the bags under my eyes and then use rouge and lipstick to hide how pale and drawn my face looks, people might think that the author of *How to Be Sick* isn't sick. On the other hand, there will be so many people there whom I haven't seen for a long time that it will make me feel good to look good for them." This inner dialogue may sound trivial, but at the time, it was terribly stressful for me. In the end, I compromised and put on some lipstick.

The question of how to "present" to others is especially a dilemma during the holidays and at family gatherings. If we try to look our best for everyone, we may look so good that we'll be criticized for not pitching in more with the preparations and the cleanup. The alternative is to stay in our sweats, but this can lead to feelings of guilt that we're not making an effort to look good around others.

Healthy people tend to assume it's all or nothing: people are either sick or they're not; they're either in pain or they're not. As a result, if they see us doing anything "normal," they assume we're 100 percent well. As I note in other chapters, this has happened to me many times. Someone will see me at an espresso place with a friend and assume I've recovered, unaware that I came from the bed and will collapse back onto it after the visit. People aren't deliberately being insensitive. They just don't know.

Do we push our body to the limit, or do we always play it safe?

One item on chapter 2's not-to-do list for the chronically ill was not to ignore your body's pleas to say no to an activity. I also indicated that there may be exceptions to this rule. Deciding when it would be skillful and self-compassionate to make that exception is one of the toughest choices we face.

Sometimes the desire to be like healthy people is so strong, I rebel and talk myself into pushing my body to do what it cannot reasonably do. A few years ago, my granddaughter Cam was visiting. I was so frustrated by always feeling sick when she was here that I decided to "act healthy." We have a park next door to our house. I took her there for over an hour, helping her with the slides and pushing her on the swings. I was in a defiant mood: "I'm tired of being sick. I'm just going to act as if I'm healthy." Ah, the perils of pretending. What I got for my effort was three days in bed with exacerbated symptoms. In retrospect, the skillful choice would have been to listen to my body and not go to the park. Cam wouldn't have minded. We could have played Go Fish on my bed instead.

However, sometimes a special occasion arises, and we might decide that pushing our bodies to the limit is worth the payback. In that case, for the good of our emotional well-being, the compassionate choice may be not to play it safe. In April of 2014, I agreed to go on a short vacation to a beach cottage that's about an hour and forty-five minutes from our home. Our son Jamal, his wife Bridgett, and our granddaughter Cam planned to join us there. This was a big trip for me; I rarely leave town because flu-like symptoms keep me from being out of bed for too long.

The exertion it took to pack for the trip, followed by riding in the car and then unpacking once we arrived at the cottage, pushed my body way beyond its limit. As a result, I spent most of the four days of the vacation trying to recover from the activities involved in getting there and settling in. I tried to hide how sick I felt, although my family has been around me long enough that they knew anyway.

Still, they sensed that I didn't want my illness to be the focus of the trip and so, taking their cue from me, we didn't talk about it.

During the daytime, I let myself by guided by the caring attention of mindfulness. This meant listening to my body, and so, when the family went down to the beach, except on the last day, I stayed behind to rest in bed. Despite these precautions, after we returned home, my body collapsed for a week, as if it had been doing its best to hold me together for the four days, but couldn't do it for one more minute.

The trip and the recovery afterward were a tremendous strain on my body, but I don't regret going. It was a rare opportunity to spend extended time with my son and his family, even though I know they'd have understood if I'd said I couldn't come.

I made this decision freely and fully aware of what I was getting into. But it was a tough choice.

Finally, on a lesser scale, I also think it's skillful to gently push our limits now and then so that we don't fall into a set pattern; our bodies can become so accustomed to a strict regime that we lose the ability to be flexible. For example, if I always nap at noon sharp, then if I'm fifteen minutes late one day, I feel like I'm going to collapse on the spot. So I purposefully vary the exact time I nap so that my body doesn't become conditioned to following a rigid schedule. That said, my ability to be flexible has its limits: I don't have the luxury to just skip the nap. I find this constant assessing and adjusting of my schedule to be mentally exhausting. I do it anyway, because I believe it's beneficial to my overall health.

What kind of end-of-life choices should we make?

Many people have written to me about this dilemma. Like me, they worry about finding themselves in a hospital with doctors and staff who don't understand—or don't believe—how chronically ill they are. How should we plan for the tough choices we may have to face regarding end-of-life treatment? We'd do well to plan ahead—talk to family, talk to our doctors, draw up an advance directive and have it made into a medical order signed by a doctor—so that as little as possible is left to chance.

I've used the word "exhausting" multiple times in this chapter. It's no surprise that physical and mental exhaustion are consequences of having to continually assess, evaluate, and choose a course of action while already struggling with chronic illness. Mindfulness can help here. We can remind ourselves to pay attention *with care* to the pros and cons of each choice. That will slow us down, making it more likely that we'll choose the alternative that's most beneficial and compassionate for us at the moment.

8

The Many Benefits of Patience

When we develop patience, we find that we develop
a reserve of calm and tranquility.

—THE DALAI LAMA

BEING CHRONICALLY ILL involves being *a patient*. In my experience, one of the essential mental qualities for finding a measure of peace with being a patient is *being patient*.

After I became ill, my life-long habitual reaction to delay, difficulty, or annoyance did not serve me well. I'd get angry, or at
least irritated—two distinctive features of impatience. My inability
to tolerate delay at the doctor's office, my difficulty coping with
unpleasant bodily symptoms, and my annoyance at not being
able to regain my health made my new life harder to bear. I found
myself face to face with that stark reality: a lot of the time, we
simply do not get our way. And yet it's not the fact that we don't
get our way that makes us miserable; it's how we respond to that
fact. The question becomes, do we get angry and upset, or do we
tolerate and accept whatever's happening that we don't like?

Several years ago, I began to make a conscious effort to tolerate and accept delay, difficulty, and annoyance. In other words, I began to practice being patient. I immediately noticed two things. First, being patient was a way of treating myself with compassion. Compassion is an act of reaching out to those who are suffering—including ourselves. I definitely suffer when I'm impatient. I can feel the stress in both my mind and my body. And so learning to be patient is a way of taking care of myself, which is the essence of self-compassion. Second, I noticed that being patient gave rise to equanimity—the even-tempered, peaceful state of mind that accepts with kind understanding that our lives will not always conform to our preferences.

Seeing the correlations between patience and enhanced self-compassion and between patience and equanimity convinced me that this was a mental state I should cultivate. I began to practice patience by using a four-step approach from my book *How to Wake Up*. It's a mindfulness practice for working with stressful and painful emotions.

Here are the four steps:

- ▸ Recognize it.
- ▸ Label it.
- ▸ Investigate it.
- ▸ Let it be.

Recognize that impatience has arisen.

This may take practice. You may not recognize that you're impatient because when things aren't going your way, there's a tendency to think that the cause of any anger or upset you're feeling is external to you. While it's true that what's going on externally may not be to your liking—it may not even be fair—impatience as a response is not coming from "out there." It's coming from your own mind.

So start by setting the intention to watch for impatience arising in your mind as a response to things not going your way. You may know some of your triggers already: being put on hold for a long time, getting stuck in a long line, struggling to figure out a computer problem, facing an extended wait at the doctor's office, having to listen to someone take an interminably long time to explain something simple (this last one is a trait of mine that tests my own family's patience!).

In my life, I've noticed that impatience arises when people or the environment don't conform to my expectations, even in circumstances over which I have no control (for example, how long I have to wait to see a doctor). I can think of four ways in which expectations can be out of sync with reality; all four can be triggers for impatience.

First, we tend to think that the environment around us should conform to our expectations: no traffic jams, no absence of parking spaces near our destination, no long lines, no airport delays, no waiting too long for food to arrive at a restaurant.

Second, we tend to think that people should conform to our expectations. They ought to behave the way we think they *should* behave. "That woman ahead of me in the checkout line should not be making small talk with the cashier." "If he said he'd phone at 3:00, he should phone at 3:00." Even if we're "right" (it is polite, after all, to call at the time you say you will), the fact remains that people often don't live up to our expectations.

Third, our expectations are often unrealistic when it comes to mastering new skills, whether it's taking up a new craft or figuring out a new computer application or learning a new language. We expect to be able to master new skills quickly, no matter how foreign or difficult they are.

Fourth, our expectations are almost always unrealistic when it comes to what goes on in our minds. We think we should be able to control what thoughts and what emotions arise. The truth is, however, unwelcome thoughts and emotions pop up all the time. It's the nature of the mind to think and to emote; there's no stopping it. Certainly being impatient doesn't put a stop to it!

Try to come up with concrete examples from your own life that fit into these four categories of expectations. This alone can help you recognize that you're responding to something or someone with impatience.

Label impatience when it is present in your mind.

The purpose of using a label is to hold impatience in your awareness so that you can investigate it. The key to successful labeling is to do it nonjudgmentally; it's hard to investigate an emotion if you're blaming yourself for its presence. You might say one of the following silently or softly to yourself:

- ▸ "Feeling impatient."
- ▸ "Impatience has arisen."
- ▸ "Mind filled with impatience."

Investigate how impatience feels in your mind and in your body.

Get to know how impatience feels. Is your mind calm or agitated? Is your body relaxed or tensed? I have yet to experience impatience as pleasant, either in my mind or my body. And the realization that it feels unpleasant helps motivate me to try and change the way I respond when I'm faced with setbacks or annoyances. Allowing yourself to truly feel the impatience is important because you can't begin to transform a stressful mental state until you accept that you're caught up in it.

Continuing with your investigation, try some strategies for

transforming impatience into patience. Start with those times when your environment or the people around you aren't conforming to your expectations. Perhaps you're stuck in a traffic jam or you find yourself behind that person in the checkout line who's chatting with the cashier. Notice if you're responding with impatience; if you are, try labeling it.

Next, turn your attention to how impatience feels in your mind and in your body. Then ask yourself, "Is there anything I can do to change the situation that won't make matters worse for myself or others?" If the answer is no (which it almost always will be), then see if you can find something enjoyable about it by directing your attention to something pleasant or interesting to focus on while you wait the situation out.

This is a mindfulness practice because you're making a conscious choice to turn your attention away from the impatience in your mind and onto something else in your field of awareness. When I feel impatience arise, I can almost always find something in my present-moment experience that arouses my curiosity or interest. This can transform impatience into patience.

If you're in a traffic jam, that "enjoyable something" might be looking at the different makes and models of the cars around you; it might be beginning to chat with another person in the car; it might be finding a radio station to listen to. If I'm in that check-out line, it might be noticing with amusement the ridiculous headlines on those sensational magazines that sit in racks at the cashier stand; it might be looking at the people around me—how everyone looks different and has a whole life story of his or her own that I know nothing about; it might even be eavesdropping on the content of the chatter that's holding me up!

In fact, I try to cultivate friendliness toward those chatterers—to enjoy how they're enjoying each other's company. After all, what's another minute or two in line? If, like me, you have trouble standing for long, you can look for something to lean on or take a wide stance with your legs so you're better balanced. Sometimes I bring a cane.

My point is that, yes, your first choice may be to institute a "no traffic jam on the freeway" rule and a "no chatting at the checkout counter" directive, but most of the time in life, we don't get our first choice. When this happens, if the alternatives are to get upset and angry, or to find a way to make the experience enjoyable, or at least tolerable—I know which one feels better to me.

Let's move to those unrealistic expectations regarding the mastery of a new skill. Investigating your impatience is likely to reveal that your assumption that you should immediately become competent partially stems from your cultural conditioning to hurry, hurry, hurry, no matter what you're doing. If you were to make a conscious effort to be patient and proceed more slowly, not only might you enjoy yourself more, but you're likely to do a better job of mastering the skill in question.

Finally, there's that out-of-touch-with-reality expectation that you should be able to control what goes on in your mind. Instead of getting impatient (that is, angry or upset) about unwelcome thoughts and emotions, you can work on holding them more lightly—sometimes even with a wry smile as you reflect on your mind's seemingly nonstop unruliness. Doing this is a compassionate response to what arises in the mind.

Let it be.

The odds are good that at this point in your investigation, you're well on your way to transforming impatience into patience. Then you can take the last step in the four-step approach: letting impatience be.

Transforming painful and stressful emotions takes practice

and... patience! In one of the first Buddhist books I ever read, *Mindfulness in Plain English*, Bhante Gunaratana says this about the mind:

> [Sometime] you will come face to face with the sudden and shocking realization that you are completely crazy. Your mind is a shrieking, gibbering madhouse on wheels barreling pell-mell down the hill, utterly out of control and hopeless. No problem.

I love this quotation for two reasons. First, I find it reassuring to know that I'm not alone in having a shrieking, gibbering, madhouse on wheels for a mind. Second, Bhante says, "No problem." I take "no problem" to mean that I can learn to be patient with this "crazy" mind. If I'm still feeling impatient after I've investigated what's going on, I *let it be* by calmly accepting the presence of impatience, knowing that, with time, conditions will change... and so will my mind.

I hope you'll practice being patient. Learning how to be patient has helped me find a measure of peace with being chronically ill. It's the peace of mind that comes with accepting, without aversion, that delays, difficulties, and annoyances will inevitably be among life's experiences. I still do get impatient sometimes. When this happens, I try to remember to be patient with my impatience. That's the compassionate way to treat our inability to always respond the way we wish we could.

9

Cultivating Kindness

People will forget what you said, people will
forget what you did, but people will never
forget how you made them feel.

—MAYA ANGELOU

KINDNESS IS ONE of my favorite words. I associate it with the phrase *in kind*—that is, "in the same way"—meaning that when we're being kind, we're treating others in the same way we hope they'll treat us. When I think of the people in my life whom I like to be around the most, the one quality they share is that they're kind. They may be high-powered professionals; they may be utility workers in my neighborhood. The quality they share—and that I treasure—is kindness. I treasure it because what Maya Angelou said is true: I never forget how they made me feel.

Kindness is a universal form of communication. All it asks of us is that we be friendly, caring, and considerate. Many years ago, as a favor to a friend, my husband and I spent an afternoon visiting her mother who was alone in San Francisco. Our friend's mother was from Argentina and spoke no English. We spoke no Spanish. She made us tea and showed us some pictures. We responded with smiles. Beyond that, the only means of communication available to us was kindness. There were long periods of time when the three of us simply sat, looking at each other with friendliness and care. It was a rich and fulfilling experience. Whenever I recall that afternoon, I see her kind face, and a warm feeling arises in my heart.

Kindness is a quality of mind that we can cultivate toward ourselves, as well as others. Many of us struggle to treat ourselves kindly. Having been conditioned throughout our lives to hold ourselves to impossible standards, we've become our own harshest critics. If you're quick to direct negative judgment at yourself, pause for a moment and imagine how it would feel if you spent the entire day being friendly, caring, and considerate to yourself.

If you can imagine it, you can do it. No matter how deeply ingrained your conditioning, you can change. As noted in chapter 5, the Buddha taught—and modern neuroscientists are confirming—that the mind is flexible and changeable. This means that, in the same way that you can change how you respond to the Want Monster, you can learn to be friendly, caring, and considerate to yourself.

To begin cultivating kindness, it's helpful to see what others have said about it. Here's a collection of quotations, followed by my reflections.

My religion is very simple. My religion is kindness.
—THE FOURTEENTH DALAI LAMA

Although the words "kindness" and "compassion" are often used interchangeably, there's a difference between them. Compassion arises when we reach out to help a person who is suffering and unhappy. By contrast, kindness is the simple act of being friendly, caring, and considerate toward those we meet, whether they're suffering or not. In my book *How to Wake Up*, I describe what I call *friendliness practice.*

Here's how it works. When I leave the house, I resolve to be friendly to everyone I see, including people I don't know. I look at each person who comes into view and silently say "May you have a lovely day" or "I hope this day will be fun for you." I wish for them whatever feels natural to me at the moment. When I first look at someone, if a negative judgment begins to arise (it's amazing how easily we can judge people we don't even know), I immediately direct a friendly thought toward that person. Invariably, the judgment disappears.

I devised this practice so that I could turn being kind into a habit—or, as the Dalai Lama put it, into my religion.

Tenderness and kindness are not signs of weakness and despair, but manifestations of strength and resolution.
—KAHLIL GIBRAN

Kindness to another person, even if we only offer a heartfelt smile, takes us out of being preoccupied with our own lives. We spend a good part of our time lost in our personal stories. They may be about the past or about some imagined future, or they may even be a running commentary about what's going on in the present. It takes strength and resolution to drop our self-focused thinking and turn our attention to how we might make another person's day a bit brighter.

Kindness is within our power even when fondness is not.
—SAMUEL JOHNSON

This reminds me of a quotation from the Buddha that is often misstated this way: "Hatred does not cease by hatred, but only by love." The written record of his teaching, however, indicates that he put it this way: "Hatred does not cease by hatred, but only by nonhatred." To me, this second version is more realistic. There are some people whom I find hard to love. Nevertheless, I've come to realize that when I direct hatred at them, I'm the one who suffers. So I cultivate nonhatred for them. In other words, I cultivate kindness.

To do this, I start by recognizing that we're not so different. Like me, they want to be happy and free from suffering. It's true that I may not want to hang out with them; even so, being friendly, caring, and considerate toward them turns out to be an act of kindness, not just toward them but toward me too, because harboring thoughts of hatred and ill-will always make me feel bad.

I've always depended on the kindness of strangers.
—BLANCHE IN TENNESSEE WILLIAMS'S *A Streetcar Named Desire*

In the context of Williams's play, Blanche's comment is sad and heartbreaking. But when I unexpectedly found myself surrounded by strangers during the traumatic years when my husband was taking me from medical facility to medical facility in a desperate attempt to find a diagnosis for my illness, I came to depend on the kindness of strangers to help get me through emotionally—a fellow patient in the waiting room who gave me a friendly smile, a lab technician who cared about my comfort. Their behavior, in turn, helped teach me to be kind to strangers.

Kindness can become its own motive.
We are made kind by being kind.
—ERIC HOFFER

This quotation echoes another of the Buddha's teachings—how our actions become the inclination of our minds. Both the Buddha and Hoffer are saying that each act of kindness strengthens our inclination to be kind again. We're planting a behavioral seed that can grow into a habit. I like to think of it as building a kindness muscle.

Be kind to people whether they deserve your kindness or not.
If your kindness reaches the deserving, good for you; if your
kindness reaches the undeserving, take joy in your compassion.
—JAMES FADIMAN AND ROBERT FRAGER

As kindness becomes a habit, we stop engaging in the mental gymnastics of making sure that someone really and truly deserves our kindness before we dole it out. Wouldn't it feel great if kindness became our natural response to others as we made our way through life? I know it would feel great to me.

No act of kindness, no matter how small, is ever wasted.
—AESOP

Another saying attributed to the Buddha expresses a similar theme: "Drop by drop is the water pot filled. Likewise, the wise man, gathering it little by little, fills himself with good." In other words, *every drop counts*, so don't stop being kind just because you can't fill that water pot with a power hose!

Here's another quotation that sounds this same theme:

Do your little bit of good where you are; it's those little
bits of good put together that overwhelm the world.
—DESMOND TUTU

I'll let Henry James have the final words on cultivating kindness:

*Three things in human life are important: the first is
to be kind; the second is to be kind; and the third is to be kind.*

II. Mindfulness: Potent Medicine for Easing the Symptoms of Chronic Illness

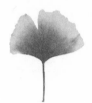

10

Mindfulness Can Ease Physical Suffering
by Easing Mental Suffering

Nothing in life is to be feared, it is only to be understood.
—MARIE CURIE

MINDFULNESS IS the practice of turning your attention with care to your experience of the moment. *With care* means paying attention with kindness, friendliness, and compassion. Without that element of care, it's easy to resist any attempt to become aware of what's going on in your mind and in your body, particularly if what's going on is not pleasant.

Let's face it, the present moment is not always a pleasant moment. If you have a migraine or if you're in a serious disagreement with someone at a medical clinic, being in the moment is not a joyful experience. In other words, mindfulness is not necessarily synonymous with joy. That said, paying caring attention to physical discomfort and to mental stress *can* help you make peace with your life as it is at the moment.

Making peace starts with gently acknowledging what's going

on: "My poor head is hurting" or "Disagreeing with this person does not feel good, but it's what's happening right now, so I'll see it through as calmly as I can." The alternative to acknowledging your experience is to turn away from it in aversion. This tends to make matters worse by increasing your dissatisfaction and frustration with your circumstances as they are. So always try to bring an attitude of self-compassion to your mindfulness practice.

Mindfulness can be practiced inside or outside of meditation. Here's the basic practice: stop for a few seconds and, with an attitude of care for yourself and for how you're feeling, take three or four conscious breaths, paying attention to the physical sensation of the breath as it comes in and goes out of your body. The sensation of the breath is a good anchor, because it's a sensation that's always taking place in the present moment. With practice, you can learn to keep your attention on your experience of the moment by using this simple conscious breathing technique. The more you practice, the easier it becomes.

In the next three chapters, I invite you to explore how mindfulness practice can help ease the physical discomfort that accompanies chronic pain and illness.

The Three Components of Physical Discomfort

It may surprise you to learn that physical discomfort is not just the result of what's going on in your body. It has three components:

- ▸ The unpleasant physical sensation itself (pain, aching muscles, fatigue).
- ▸ Your emotional reaction to that discomfort (frustration, irritation, fear).
- ▸ The thoughts that are related to the first two components. These are the stress-filled stories you tell yourself—and

then believe without question—such as "This pain will never go away."

Note that two of the three components that make up your experience of physical discomfort are mental in origin. These two mental components are often referred to as "mental suffering." They can make your physical discomfort worse because mental reactions are responded to and felt in the body.

This chapter explores the second and third components of physical discomfort: stressful emotions and stressful thought patterns. It covers how mindfulness of these two components can keep physical symptoms from becoming worse. The next chapter describes several mindfulness practices that address physical discomfort itself. The last chapter in this section contains instructions for practicing mindfulness meditation.

Stressful Emotions

When physical symptoms are intense, your mind can feel like a muddy blur. This makes it difficult to identify what emotions are present in your mind at the moment. With caring attentiveness, however, the "mud" can settle, making it possible to identify those emotions: "I'm frustrated"; "Irritation is present"; "This is what fear feels like."

To help that mud settle, follow the basic instructions for mindfulness practice: with an attitude of care for yourself and for how you're feeling, take several conscious breaths, turning your attention to the physical sensation of the breath as it comes in and goes out of your body. Now, also observe what emotions are present in your mind. This is one of the most beneficial functions of mindfulness: it helps you identify what's going on in your mind, such as frustration, irritation, or fear.

Mindfulness also helps you respond skillfully to those emotions.

This can ease both your mental and physical suffering. Here's how this works. Once you recognize the presence of a stressful emotion, there are two ways to respond. You can respond with aversion or you can respond with acceptance. Let's look at the first choice.

When you react with aversion to a stressful emotion, you're resisting what's going on in your mind. It's as if you're saying to the emotion, "Go away!" You may even mount a militant battle against the emotion by trying to force it out of your mind. This kind of response increases your mental suffering because aversion to the presence of an emotion almost always has the effect of intensifying it. In addition, now you're dealing with two stressful emotions: frustration *and* aversion to the frustration; irritation *and* aversion to the irritation; fear *and* aversion to the fear.

Aversion to what's present in your mind is also likely to increase your physical suffering because stressful emotions trigger physical reactions in the body. For example, if you're in physical pain, you may respond by getting irritated. This emotional reaction can lead to tightening the muscles that surround the point of pain. The result is an increase in your overall pain load. Other common physical reactions to stressful emotions are heart racing, agitation, nausea, and fatigue.

The alternative to responding with aversion is to respond with acceptance. As Marie Curie said in the epigraph that begins this chapter: "Nothing in life is to be feared, it is only to be understood." Sticking with the example of feeling irritated at physical pain, the way to understand and accept what's going on in your mind is to gently acknowledge that irritation is present, and then incline your mind toward kindness and compassion for yourself. After all, who doesn't get irritated at pain sometimes?

Once you begin to treat yourself with kindness, you can calmly and gently begin to examine the actual physical discomfort. That's the subject of the next chapter. Suffice it to say here that a physical sensation is not the solid block of discomfort that you might think it is. Physical discomfort is made up of multiple sensations that are constantly changing. This reflection can help you remember that your frustration is impermanent too. It arose, and it will pass. This recognition alone can keep it from intensifying, which will, of course, ease your mental suffering and, perhaps, your physical suffering too.

Stressful Thought Patterns

Unpleasant physical sensations and the stressful emotions that accompany them tend to trigger stressful thought patterns— full-blown stories about your life that have little or no basis in fact. Some typical stressful thoughts that accompany physical discomfort are "This pain will never go away" and "I'll never feel well enough to leave the house again."

You may not even stop there. You might keep spinning these stories until you're telling yourself "I've ruined my partner's life" or "No one cares about my pain." As with stressful emotions, stressful thought patterns tend to trigger physical reactions in the body, such as a racing heart and tightening muscles.

To become aware of the stories you're telling yourself about your physical discomfort, once again, with an attitude of care for yourself, take several conscious breaths, paying attention to the physical sensation of the breath as it comes in and goes out of your body. This time, as you do it, try to observe what stressful thought patterns are running through your mind. This may not be easy: thoughts have a tendency to skitter away when you try and look directly at them.

Becoming mindfully aware of the stories you spin gives you the opportunity to make a conscious choice. You can continue to believe them, or you can calmly assess their validity. Are you sure you've ruined your partner's life or that no one cares about your pain? Early on in my illness, I believed both these thoughts, neither of which turned out to be true.

At a meditation retreat in the 1990s, Buddhist nun Ayya Khema said to us, "Most thoughts are just rubbish, but we believe them anyway." It took several years of chronic illness for me to recognize that I was causing myself undue mental suffering by spinning stressful stories about my physical discomfort and then accepting them as true without question simply because I had thought them. Mindfulness practice was the principal tool that helped me realize what I was doing.

Mindful attention calms and steadies the mind, giving you breathing room to reflect and to respond more skillfully to the stressful emotions and the stressful thought patterns that tend to accompany physical discomfort. Not only can this ease your mental suffering, it can also ease your physical suffering because stressful thoughts and emotions are felt physically in the body. As the wonderfully blunt Zen teacher Joko Beck said: "What makes life so frightening is that we let ourselves be carried away in the garbage of our whirling minds. We don't have to do that."

II

Mindfulness Practices That Address Physical Discomfort

If we practice mindfulness, we always have
a place to be when we're afraid.

—THICH NHAT HANH

To REITERATE a point from the previous chapter, physical discomfort has three components: the unpleasant physical sensation itself, the emotional reaction to it, and the thought patterns that are related to the first two components. This chapter focuses on practices that can address the unpleasant physical sensations themselves.

Two preliminary notes.

If pain is one of your symptoms, I want to be clear from the outset that I don't have a negative view of pain medication. Taking medication for pain is not a sign of weakness. Many of us have been told repeatedly "No pain, no gain" and "Push through the pain." I suspect that people who offer this advice have never suffered from chronic pain themselves. Everyone has to find what's right for his or her body. For many people, it's a combination of pain medication and the practices I'm about to describe.

Second, with each of these practices, find a comfortable position—sitting or lying down—and begin by breathing mindfully. By this I mean take a minute or two, and pay caring attention to the physical sensation of the breath as it comes in and goes out of your body. As you're doing this, do a quick scan of your body from head to toe. If you feel muscles that are tight, see if they might relax under your caring attention. If not, that's fine. When you're ready, try one of the following mindfulness practices and see if it helps relieve your physical discomfort. Over time, I hope you'll experiment with each of them to find out which ones work for you.

Focus on the physical discomfort itself, paying careful attention to the sensations that make it up.

People who are chronically ill often come to see their bodies as the enemy. In the first few years of my illness, I certainly did. Out of ignorance, I'd separated my mind from my body, and it was "me" against "it." This perception that the body is the enemy gives rise to stressful emotions, such as frustration and fear. It can even give rise to anger—that conviction that you've been wronged. As discussed in the previous chapter, these emotions themselves often trigger bodily reactions that can lead to new symptoms or to the intensification of existing ones.

By focusing your attention on the physical discomfort itself, instead of on your stories about it, this first mindfulness practice unites your mind and your body so that you stop seeing your body as a separate entity that's purposefully causing you discomfort.

Your body may be struggling, but it's doing the best it can to support you and to sustain life.

You can begin this practice by turning your attention to a point of discomfort in your body. You're going to examine it with caring attentiveness. Is there burning? Is there throbbing? Tingling? Pressure? Heat? Cold? Are there waves of sensations in which the discomfort gets more intense and then less intense? Study your discomfort, becoming as familiar with it as a scientist examining a new phenomenon.

This separating out of sensations is called "sensory splitting." It helps you see that what you've been thinking of as a permanent solid block of physical discomfort, such as pain, is actually many different constantly changing sensations. When you distinguish the sensations in this manner, physical discomfort is no longer "a thing," and so you're much less likely to be carried away by stress-filled thoughts about it, such as "This discomfort will never go away."

It can even help to drop the words you usually use to identify the discomfort—words such as "pain" or "fatigue"—and simply be aware of the physical sensations themselves as arising and passing experiences in your body. Doing this helps you see the impermanent nature of the various physical sensations that are part of your physical discomfort.

End this practice by bringing an attitude of kindness toward your entire body. Treat it the way you'd treat a child who is suffering, reaching out with care and compassion. Your body is so much more than the physical discomfort you're experiencing. Making friends with this remarkable organism is emotionally calming and healing. It can release tension in your body, which, in itself, can ease your physical discomfort.

Rest your attention on a symptom-free part of your body.

In this mindfulness practice, you turn your attention to a symptom-free part of your body. At first, you might think there isn't such a place, but with patience and persistence, you can find it. It could be your toes or your face or your chest. Relax into that symptom-free feeling, allowing it to become the predominant sensation in your experience—even if for just a few moments. This allows you to see that you are not *just* physical discomfort, since there's at least one place on your body that is symptom-free.

You can take this technique a step further and engage a symptom-free area in some movement. I'll reveal a secret of mine—since you won't see me in action. I sometimes lie on my back in bed and move my hands in balletic movements. I love to watch my hands and fingers imitate the grace of a ballerina.

This idea came from Buddhist teacher Mary Orr at a meditation retreat many years ago. At the retreat, we alternated periods of sitting and walking meditation. In the latter, the instruction was to walk very slowly, staying mindfully aware of the physical sensation of one foot touching the ground as the other foot came off the ground. I was having terrible back pain and found it too hard to engage in walking meditation. I felt like my whole being had narrowed and become "back pain," so I sought the help of a teacher.

Mary told me to lie down during the walking period and be mindfully aware of the physical sensation of my hands moving in the air. Little did I know the joy this would bring; I wound up playing "Itsy Bitsy Spider" for the rest of the retreat—mindfully, of course! I doubt that this is what Mary had in mind but, in addition to having fun, I learned that my body was not just a painful back.

Consciously pay attention to something pleasant or at least interesting in your field of awareness.

Turn your attention to as many things other than your pain or discomfort as you can—the sight and feel of the sun shining through the window, the sound of cars passing by, a fleeting thought about what you'll eat for dinner, the hum of the refrigerator motor, the physical sensation of a wisp of hair on your cheek, an odor coming from the kitchen. Paying attention to a variety of sensory inputs eases physical discomfort because it relegates it to just one of the many sensory experiences going on in the moment.

Use imagery to transport yourself to a pleasant place.

Think of a special place you've been to or would like to visit. Close your eyes and make its image vivid in your mind. My place is Maké Horse Beach on the island of Molokai. I was there many times before I became chronically ill, so it's easy for me to recall its turquoise water, the sound of surf crashing on the rocks, the hot sand on my skin, the saltwater air. Using imagery to take your mind off your physical discomfort relaxes the body, and this may help ease your symptoms.

Describe your present-moment experience.

This is a mindfulness practice that my daughter Mara introduced me to. It comes from a remarkable teacher named Byron Katie whom we'll encounter again in chapter 13, "Breaking Free from Stressful Thinking Patterns." I altered the practice from Katie's original so it could be used specifically to help with physical discomfort. The basic practice is to ground yourself in the present by describing, in a neutral fashion, what is happening in your life at this moment. For example, you might say to yourself "Lying on a bed, with shoulder pain" or "Sitting in a waiting-room chair, feeling sick."

The key is to describe what you're experiencing without using emotionally charged words that can intensify your symptoms. In my first example, by saying "Lying on a bed, with shoulder pain," you're simply acknowledging that your shoulder is in pain. Compare this to saying "Lying on a bed, with *relentless* shoulder pain." In my second example, by saying "Sitting in a waiting-room chair, feeling sick," you're simply acknowledging the sick feeling without adding an emotional dimension, such as "Sitting in a waiting-room chair, feeling *unbearably* sick."

Leaving out these emotionally charged words makes it much less likely that you'll start spinning stressful thoughts about the physical discomfort, such as "I hate this pain. I'm stuck with it: it will never go away." In addition, by neutrally describing what you happen to be experiencing at the moment, you're not setting the physical discomfort in stone. You're leaving the door open for change. No matter how unpleasant physical discomfort is, it could change at any moment. Pain is not always relentless. Sick feelings are not always unbearable.

Although it requires discipline on my part, I take up this practice whenever I realize that I've added emotional distress to my physical symptoms by including descriptors, such as "relentless," "horrible," or "unbearable"—words that lead me to believe that the unpleasant sensation is here to stay. But it never is. Everything changes.

Notice how your body breathes on its own.

Sometimes this instruction is given as part of formal meditation practice. I use it as a mindfulness technique to help soothe my body when I'm experiencing unpleasant physical sensations. It's particularly helpful when I first lie down to rest or nap, because that's when I become more acutely aware of bodily discomfort.

To try this technique, turn your attention to the physical sensation of the breath as it comes in and goes out of your body. Breathe gently, without exerting any effort to control the length of the in- or the out-breath. As you're doing this, you might try counting each breath up to whatever number feels comfortable, be it five or fifty, and then start over. Or, as you breathe, you could silently say "in" and "out."

Counting breaths or using the words "in" and "out" helps keep your mind from wandering off into thoughts or stressful stories about bodily discomfort. If your mind does wander off, when you become aware it's happened, without judgment, return to counting breaths or silently repeating "in" and "out."

When I practice this, after a few minutes, I can feel a calming effect on whatever bodily discomfort I'm experiencing at the moment. The calming comes from not asking anything of my body. I'm simply letting it breathe at its own pace, without interfering.

Practice the body scan.

The body scan is a mindfulness practice in which you move your attention from one part of your body to another, simply noticing the physical sensations present at the moment. As you move to each new area, linger there and imagine that you're breathing into it and out of it. After some moments, you mentally let go of that area and move your attention to the next.

As you practice this, you may not feel any sensations in some parts of your body. That's fine; just note, "not feeling anything in particular." Or you may feel pain or another unpleasant sensation. In this case, as you breathe into that part of your body, try to allow any tension associated with it to release itself. The tension may be in your mind, in your body, or in both. If you can't release the tension, then try to let it soften by simply letting the unpleasant sensation be as it is without attaching a negative judgment or any meaning to it. It's just a sensation, and sensations are impermanent.

Throughout the exercise, be sure you're giving your body *caring* attention. Even though your illness may make you feel as if your body has let you down, in reality, it's working hard for you. Let go of any expectations or wishes; in other words, don't have any particular results in mind. Simply set the intention to be with your body with curiosity and kindness.

I suggest that you read through all the instructions before starting. You could even record them and play them back as you do the exercise.

1. Find a comfortable place to lie down where you won't be disturbed. (In my opinion, if lying down causes you to fall sleep, that's a bonus for your body!) Put aside anywhere from twenty to fifty minutes for the scan. The time you allot will affect the speed at which you move from one area of your body to another.

2. Close your eyes and rest your attention on the physical sensation of your breath as it comes in and goes out of your body. Breathing in, know you're breathing in. Breathing out, know you're breathing out. As you do this, feel that your body is connected to whatever is solid beneath it.

3. Move your attention to the toes of your left foot. Imagine you're breathing into your toes and out from your toes. This may take some practice. It helps to imagine your breath flowing from the in-breath at your nostrils, down through your body, and into your toes. Feel any sensations in your toes, or note the lack of sensation. If you feel tension in your toes or in your mind, see if directing caring attention to it enables it to release some. If it doesn't, gently let it be, always with an attitude of kindness and compassion for your discomfort. If your attention wanders off into thoughts, gently bring your attention back to your left toes.

4. When you're ready, on the out-breath, mentally leave your toes and move your attention to the sole of your left foot, then to the heel, and then to the ankle, following the same instructions as for the toes.

5. Following the same instructions, move your attention through the different areas of your body in this order:

- The lower left leg, including the calf, the shin, the knee
- The left thigh—front and back—and its connection to the left hip
- The right toes, the sole of the foot, the heel, the ankle, the calf, the shin, the knee, the thigh, the connection of the thigh to the right hip
- The pelvic region and its organs
- The abdominal region and the organs of the digestive system
- The tailbone and then up the back from the lower to the middle to the upper back
- The chest, including the heart, the lungs, and the breasts
- The fingertips of your left hand, the back of the hand, the palm, the wrist, the forearm, the elbow, the upper arm
- The fingertips of your right hand, the back of the hand, the palm, the wrist, the forearm, the elbow, the upper arm
- The shoulders and armpits, up into the neck
- The jaw and then the teeth, the tongue, the mouth, and the lips
- The cheeks and sinuses, the eyes, the muscles around the eyes, the forehead, the temples, the ears
- The back of the scalp up to the top of the head

6. To finish the exercise, shift your attention back to the sensation

of your breath and, once again, become aware of your body as a whole, alive from head to toe with physical sensations. Send caring and kind thoughts to this remarkable organism that works so hard to support and sustain you.

Be patient as you explore this set of mindfulness practices. If you try one and it isn't helpful, that's fine. Simply say to yourself with kindness, "That one's not for me. I'll try another one."

12

Formal Mindfulness Meditation Can Help Your Mind Help Your Body

You don't have to clear your mind. You just give your mind a chance to clear itself.

—AJAHN CHAH

I THINK OF MEDITATION practice as the opportunity to sit (or lie) down and observe your mind. It's not about putting an end to thinking. Who can do that? I certainly can't. Becoming aware of what's going on in your mind can be a challenge; to be frank, it's not always a pretty sight. The Tibetan Buddhist teacher Pema Chödrön draws an analogy to a lake: when the water clears, you can see the sparkling jewels at the bottom, but you also see the worn shoes and the old tires—recurring disappointment and sadness, longing and fear.

Each of you has had unique life experiences that have affected your disposition in different ways. As a result, when the mind gets quiet, for some of you, the "old tire" that pops up is anger; for others, it might be worry. After practicing meditation for a while, you start to see the habits that have been worn into the mind from past conditioning. Pema Chödrön says that meditation is like doing a PhD dissertation—but the subject is yourself.

Let your mind help your body.

Recall that physical discomfort has three components: the physical sensation itself, the emotional reaction to it, and the stories you spin about it. Formal meditation practice provides a quiet and uninterrupted setting for watching those emotional reactions and for challenging the validity of those stressful stories.

For example, if you're in physical pain, you may also feel frustrated and irritated at your body. But when you're distracted by the sights and sounds and other sensory inputs all around you—not to mention the stories about how life isn't fair, etc.—you may not even realize that these two emotions are present in your mind. You feel "off" emotionally, and you know that you're suffering mentally, but you're unable to pinpoint the specific emotions that are in play. In a meditation setting, however, there are few, if any, outside sensory distractions. As a result, it's easier to direct caring attention to what's going on in your mind. The water clears, and there they are: those worn-out shoes of frustration and irritation.

Recognizing their presence gives you the opportunity to develop some skill in responding to them. For example, once you've recognized the presence of frustration and irritation in your mind, the simple act of nonjudgmentally studying them with caring attention instead of feeding them with stressful stories, such as "I hate this pain" or "This pain will never go away," can stop them in their tracks and keep them from intensifying. This alone can ease your mental suffering.

Formal meditation also makes it easier to see that frustration and irritation are impermanent, that they are nothing more than fluid and ever-changing events in the mind. They've arisen based on causes and conditions in your life at the moment, and they'll pass out of the mind—as do all emotions. There's no reason to treat them as intrinsic features of who you are. Seeing this can help ease your mental suffering.

Both of these skillful responses to stressful emotions—nonjudgmental attention and reflections on impermanence—can ease your physical suffering. The mind and body are interconnected. Formal meditation practice can bring this into sharp focus. Physical discomfort can set off stressful emotions, such as frustration and irritation, even fear. This can lead to the spinning of stressful stories about the present and the future. In turn, these emotions and stories can increase your physical discomfort by intensifying the symptoms you're already experiencing or by triggering new symptoms, such as muscle contractions or a racing heart.

In summary, seeing what's going on in your mind can help ease your physical symptoms, and the most effective way to see what's going on in your mind is to meditate.

How to meditate.

There are many different meditation techniques. What follows is a description of the most common type of mindfulness meditation. It's helpful to have access to a teacher who can answer questions as they arise, but these instructions can get you started.

Pick a quiet place and a time when you won't be interrupted. Decide ahead of time how long you'll meditate; otherwise your mind is likely to come up with any number of excuses to stop if you're finding it difficult. Find a comfortable position—sitting on the floor, in a chair, or lying down.

In choosing an amount of time and what position to be in, the most important consideration is to be flexible. Before I got sick, I had such an inflexible meditation schedule—sit upright for forty-five minutes, twice a day—that when illness prevented me from keeping to the schedule, I gave up meditation altogether, even though I'd been doing it for ten years. It took me another ten years to start practicing again. Depending on how I'm feeling, I may only set aside twenty minutes... and I always meditate lying down.

Begin by gently closing your eyes. Do a quick scan of your body, from the top of your head to your toes. Is your body tired? Is it full of energy? Is there any discomfort? The idea here is to ground your attention in your body.

Now notice the physical sensation of your breath as it comes in and goes out of your body. Find the place in your body where that physical sensation is the strongest. It might be in your nostrils or at the back of your throat. It might be in the rise and fall of the abdomen. It might be in the expansion and contraction of your entire torso. It doesn't matter. Just rest your attention on the sensations that most strongly let you know that your breath is coming in and going out of your body. You'll come back to the physical sensation of your breath at this place over and over. It will become your anchor spot to the present moment.

As you breathe, investigate the physical sensation of your breathing with interest. Notice how the in-breath feels different from the out-breath. Notice the difference in the feeling of the beginning, middle, and end of the in- and out-breaths. When you recognize that your attention has strayed from the breath to other incoming sensory data (a thought, a physical sensation, a sound), gently bring your attention back to the physical sensation of the breath going in and out of your body at your anchor spot.

Remember—whether this is your first time meditating or your ten-thousandth time, your mind will still stray from the breath! One of the beauties of meditation is that it's okay to begin again... and again and again. The whole practice can be thought of as this returning again and again, practicing this returning, slowly getting better at it.

Usually when you notice that your attention has strayed from the breath, it's easy to return to following it at your anchor spot. That said, sometimes another sensory input becomes more compelling than the breath. If that happens, let go of your focus on the breath and bring to this sensory input the same attentive quality that you brought to the breath. If it's an unpleasant physical sensation, don't attach any meaning to it; just notice the unpleasantness without judgment. When the sensory input becomes less compelling, return to the physical sensation of the breath at your anchor spot.

If it's a thought or emotion that has become so compelling that you can't keep your focus on the breath, shift your attention to the thought or emotion and just patiently watch it, study it without judgment. Get to know what it is. Thoughts and emotions come and go in the mind in an ever-changing flow. They're not solid entities or permanent features of your identity. They arise due to conditions in your life and will eventually pass on through the mind. When the thought or emotion becomes less compelling, return to following your breath at your anchor spot.

These are basic mindfulness meditation instructions: return over and over again to the physical sensation of the breath coming in and going out of your body. Wherever the meditation takes you, meet your experience with curiosity and open-heartedness, not judgment. If judgment does arise, study it as well: What's the story? Does it create its own set of physical sensations? And so on.

You can watch what's going on in your mind by practicing mindfulness outside of meditation, of course. Formal meditation practice, however, can help you become more adept at this; meditation sharpens your ability to pay attention to your present-moment experience.

Finally, it's important to point out that if you have unresolved psychological issues (for example, mistreatment by overly critical parents or an unresolved past trauma), mindfulness meditation may not be a good choice for you at this time in your life. When your mind becomes quiet and calm, repressed or charged thoughts and emotional issues can come up—issues you may have been keeping at arm's length or that you didn't even realize existed.

Mindfulness meditation is an excellent tool for seeing that you need not believe in or act upon the ever-changing array of thoughts and emotions that arise in the mind. But if these unresolved issues are part of your deeply embedded personal psychological history (as opposed to being the thoughts and emotions that typically come and go for everyone during meditation, such as a wave of sadness or worry), they can stick in your mind and increase in intensity, leading to anxiety, anxiousness, and fearfulness.

This is not a common occurrence when practicing mindfulness meditation, but if it happens to you, please don't blame yourself. Instead, with kindness and compassion toward yourself over the suffering you're experiencing, stop meditating and talk to a trusted meditation teacher (one with experience in these matters) or consult with a qualified mental health practitioner, perhaps a trauma specialist.

III. Responding Wisely to Troubling
Thoughts and Emotions

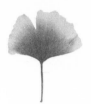

13

Breaking Free from Stressful Thinking Patterns

If you can change your mind, you can change your life.

—WILLIAM JAMES

M ANY OF US are adept at making ourselves unhappy by taking a neutral, fact-based thought, turning it into a stressful one, and then spinning that stressful thought into an even *more* stressful story. I'm quite good at this myself. I start with a harmless thought and before I'm even aware of it, I'm suffering through an elaborate stress-filled tale that may reflect my worries and fears about the future, but has no basis in reality.

To illustrate my unfortunate expertise at this, here are two neutral, fact-based thoughts that started off innocently enough for me:

- ▸ "A friend is coming over tomorrow."
- ▸ "I'm seeing a new specialist next week."

Each of these thoughts states a fact, free from emotional content. However, fueled by worry and anxiety over my health, I then turned them into stressful thoughts even though I had no additional information on which to base my conclusions:

- ▸ "My friend's visit is going to be a mistake."
- ▸ "The appointment with the specialist will be a big disappointment."

Having turned each of the neutral thoughts into stressful ones, my storytelling began:

- ▸ "My friend will stay much longer than I'm able to visit, and I'll be too embarrassed or undisciplined to tell her I need to lie down. It will take me days to recover, and I'll be angry at myself for not speaking up."
- ▸ "The specialist won't believe how sick I am. He might even treat me as if it's all in my head. And even if he does believe me, he won't want to take on a patient who has a complex illness with no easy fix."

Notice the multiple hypothetical scenarios I added to the simple facts that a friend was coming over and that I had an appointment with a new specialist: my friend will stay too long, I'll be embarrassed or lack discipline, I won't be able to tell her I have to lie down, it will take me days to recover, and I'll be angry at myself; the specialist won't believe what I tell him, he might think I'm a hypochondriac, and he wouldn't want the hassle of trying to care for me anyway. Whew. All this, and neither event has even occurred yet!

In this chapter, I want to share a powerful practice developed by a teacher (who's not Buddhist) named Byron Katie. She calls it "inquiry" or "four questions and a turnaround"; she presents questions we are to ask ourselves when we recognize that we're caught in the net of a stressful thought.

The purpose of *inquiry* is not to control what thoughts pop into our minds. The mind is going to think what it's going to think. Trying to control our thoughts is almost always a fruitless endeavor. What matters to our well-being is not what thoughts arise but how we respond to them. If we can learn to respond skillfully, we're much more likely to keep a stressful thought from turning into a full-blown stressful thinking pattern.

Here are Byron Katie's four questions:

1. Is the thought true?
2. Am I absolutely sure that it's true?
3. How do I feel when I think the thought?
4. Who would I be without the thought?

Before addressing Byron Katie's fifth step—the turnaround—I'll apply her four questions to the two stressful thoughts in my example. In writing this, I'll answer the way I would have. As you read it, try thinking of how you'd answer each question. I'll start with my friend's upcoming visit.

1. Is it true that my friend's visit is going to be a mistake? *Yes, I think it's true.*
2. Am I absolutely sure it's true? *Hmm. I guess I'm not absolutely sure. I'm not even 75 percent sure.*

Sometimes simply seeing that we're not absolutely sure that a stressful thought is true is enough to stop the thought in its tracks and keep us from turning it into a stress-filled story.

3. How do I feel when I think that my friend's visit is going to be a mistake? *I feel as if it's my fault for agreeing to let her come, and I feel even more nervous and worried about how it will go. Even worse, now I'm dreading her visit.*

In this situation, the dread is more painful than the worry, because dread carries guilt with it; I love my friend, yet here I am, dreading her visit. This definitely does not feel good!

4. Who would I be without the thought that the visit is going to be a mistake? *I'd be a person living in the present moment, with a chance to enjoy what I'm doing right now, instead of being lost in worry and anxiety about tomorrow.*

Now I'll try the same technique with the appointment with the new specialist.

1. Is it true that the appointment with the specialist will be a big disappointment? *Yes, it's true. They always are.*
2. Am I absolutely sure it's true? *Not really. I guess I was exaggerating a bit when I said "They always are."*
3. How do I feel when I think it will be a big disappointment? *I feel scared, and I feel angry. I'm scared that I'll be disregarded and that I won't be offered a treatment that might be beneficial. I'm angry that I'm sick because that's why I have to spend so much time in medical clinics.*
4. Who would I be without the thought that the appointment will be a big disappointment? *I'd be a person living in this moment instead of being lost in stressful thoughts about something that's a week away.*

Pausing to let my response to question 4 sink in is always helpful because it switches my focus to what's going on right now in my life. If I stop here though, I'm likely to drift back into stressful storytelling about an imagined future, so it's important to move on to Byron Katie's *turnaround.*

In the turnaround, we take the stressful thought and turn it around—change it—in a way that works for each of us individually. In other words, there's no one "right" turnaround. Then the instruction is to come up with three reasons why this new thought might be true.

I'll start with my friend's visit. Here's my turnaround: *My friend's visit won't be a mistake.* What are three reasons why this might be true?

1. She might be sensitive to my limitations and know not to stay too long.
2. I might feel comfortable enough around her to let her know when I need to lie down.
3. Maybe she'll tell me about a funny adventure she had, and we'll have a great time laughing together.

In coming up with reasons why the turnaround might be true, I've found that it's helpful to be creative in my thinking, even if it becomes absurd. For example, one reason could be "Maybe she'll get an upset stomach and have to leave early." This isn't exactly in the spirit of friendship, but letting my imagination run wild like this helps shake me loose from the rigid thinking pattern that I've fallen into—in this case, a pattern that has me believing there's only one possible outcome for this visit: it will turn out to be a mistake.

In sum, thinking of multiple reasons why the visit *might* go well drives home the point that there's no reason to believe the stressful thought that it's going to be a mistake. Thus, engaging in the turnaround helps me stop fretting and enables me to simply wait and see how the visit unfolds.

Now to the appointment with the new specialist. My turnaround: *The appointment will be a success.* What are three reasons why this might be true?

1. The doctor might not question how sick I am—at all!

2. The doctor might be sympathetic and understanding about my illness.
3. The doctor might see my illness as a challenge and want to try and help me.

When I reflect on the two dozen or so specialists I've seen about my illness, a few of them have been just as I described above, so why should I decide ahead of time that the appointment will be a disappointment even if the odds are against me? After all, if my stressful thought turns out to be true and the appointment *is* a disaster, it won't be because of the stressful stories I'm spinning about it! No doubt about it: my time could be better spent in the days leading up to the appointment.

Byron Katie's "four questions and a turnaround" has been a gift of inestimable value to me. It's such a relief to know that I can free myself from stressful thinking patterns by questioning the validity of the stories I spin about my life. I hope you'll give it a try.

14

When the Blues Come Calling

Sadness flies away on the wings of time.

—JEAN DE LA FONTAINE

UNLIKE OTHER stressful emotions, such as anger or frustration, I can't pinpoint what sets off the blues. One moment, I feel okay, and the next moment, I feel inexplicably melancholy. The blues don't seem to be tied to the intensity of my physical symptoms nor to other happenings in my life. In fact, I got the blues before I became chronically ill, so at least there's *something* I've brought with me from my pre-illness life!

The one thing I feel sure of? Everyone gets the blues now and then. In this chapter, I'll discuss some things that can help.

(Note that the "blues" is to be distinguished from a heavy or dark mood that goes unchanged for weeks at a time and interferes with work or personal relationships. The latter could be a sign of clinical depression, in which case you should seriously consider seeking the advice of a health care practitioner.)

Avoid "comparing mind."

We can talk ourselves into believing that we're the only ones who get the blues. Our neighbor who's always cheerful surely never gets them. Our friend who's in the "perfect" relationship definitely never does. And billionaires? They can't possibly get the blues! In reality, of course, the odds are high that all these people do. To reference the title of the Tom Robbins novel, "even cowgirls get the blues." In my experience, neither a carefree demeanor, nor a loving relationship, nor money to spare immunizes people from the blues.

It helps to remember that when we see our always-cheerful neighbor or our in-love friend, for the most part, we're only seeing their public faces. We don't know what their inner life is like. If we did, we'd see that it's not so different from our own. The Buddha pointed out that we are all subject to illness, injury, aging, and separation from those we love. No one gets a pass on this.

In addition to being subject to the inescapable vicissitudes of life, each of us has been conditioned by our life experiences in ways that often remain at a subconscious level. For example, if a parent repeatedly told us that nothing we did was good enough, we're likely to have internalized that message. Such conditioning can show itself unexpectedly at any time in the form of painful thoughts and emotions—either of which can trigger the blues.

I've learned to be okay with not knowing the source of my blues. What I do know is that they'll intensify if I engage in comparing mind by telling myself how blues-free everyone else must be.

Treat the blues with friendliness and compassion.

When the blues are particularly intense, I can feel as if I'm on the verge of tears all day. Part of the reason for this is that, although I may not be physically alone when the blues come calling, they make me feel isolated nevertheless. This calls for self-compassion, not self-judgment. Trying to force the blues away by telling myself that I shouldn't feel blue never works; this is because ordering myself not to feel a certain way almost always guarantees that I will feel exactly that way. So the best we can do when the blues come calling is to be mindfully aware that they're present and to let compassion for ourselves arise over any suffering we're experiencing as a result of their presence.

I have a strategy that sometimes catches the blues off-guard and, in doing so, disarms them: I treat them as old friends, maybe even saying silently or softly to myself: "Hello blues. Come to visit, have you?" Exposing them in this friendly way to the sunlight of awareness can reduce their intensity. I don't need to *love* those blues, but treating them with friendliness allows me to hold them more lightly until they run their course.

Sometimes I might even throw myself a short pity party, but I have to be sure I'm engaging in *pity with compassion* as opposed to *pity with aversion*. Angry pitying, such as "I hate the blues," or threatening thoughts, such as "These blues better not hang around all day," are not in the party spirit! By contrast, pity with compassion means that we're looking after our well-being even though we're feeling pity for ourselves. I sometimes say to myself (I might even whine it—this is, after all, a pity party): "It's not fair that I feel so blue on top of being sick."

A properly held pity party—one held with compassion not aversion—can help turn the confused and painful thoughts that can accompany the blues into simple sadness. And sadness can open our hearts to our mental suffering. A good test of whether a pity party is accompanied by compassion is to check and see if it feels right to stroke one arm with the hand of the other while speaking your "pity party" words.

Change the environment—physical or mental.

Doing something—anything (nonharmful of course)—can take a blue day and help us see it from a different, brighter perspective. This is not the same as trying to force the blues away. On the contrary, with a friendly attitude toward them, we're letting the blues accompany us as we change our environment. (Doing this might throw them so off-guard that they'll make a hasty exit!)

My go-to change of physical environment is to sit in the backyard for a bit. The outside air is refreshing, and the sights and sounds of the neighborhood fill my senses. It makes me feel part of the larger world around me. Sometimes I ask my husband to take me for a drive. We're fortunate that it only takes a few minutes for us to be on a country road. The scenery may only be the flat Central Valley of California, but I enjoy looking at the open sky and watching the parallel rows of crops go by.

There are many ways to change our mental environment. One of the best ways is to invite a friend over. Many years ago, my husband and I were fighting about something—I can't remember what. We both wanted to end the argument and move on with the day, yet neither one of us was willing to give in first. Then a friend unexpectedly came over for a visit. We both jumped at the opportunity to chat with her, and—just like that—we were no longer angry with each other. Our friend unknowingly changed our mental environment and, by doing so, changed our mood. A dark day became a light one.

Another way to change the mental environment is to do something that's just plain fun. For instance, I have a few movies that I watch over and over: *Groundhog Day, Best in Show, Gosford Park.* When the blues settle in, I put on one of them. The characters are like old friends, and with their company, I can patiently wait out my mood. Quite often, by the time I'm finished indulging in my little pleasureful activity, those blues have lifted and blown away.

Finally, doing something creative is a good way to change the mental environment. The activity doesn't need to be earth-shatteringly skillful or original. Some internet friends of mine have coloring books. You can get beautiful ones at reasonable prices, and crayons are still cheap. Or try journaling or singing along to music. My creative outlet is crocheting.

Even if these physical or mental changes don't magically turn a blue day into a bright day, they're a soothing balm that help make the blues manageable until they've run their course.

Remember that the blues, like all moods and emotions, are impermanent.

Reflecting on the impermanence of all mental states can keep the blues from intensifying and can also help us patiently wait them out. Because all phenomena are in constant flux, there's no reason to worry that every day from now on will be a "blue" day. I call this reflection on impermanence "Weather Practice."

Moods and emotions are as changeable and unpredictable as the weather. They blow in and they blow out. This metaphor is a helpful reminder that, like the weather pattern of the moment, the blues are subject to change. Right now, life may look gray, but at any moment a bit of brightness—maybe even a rainbow—may break through.

This reflection is tremendously helpful to me when the blues settle in like a dense fog. It reminds me that I don't know what tomorrow may bring. It very well might be something warm and welcoming.

Reach out to someone who's having a tough time.

Pema Chödrön said that sorrow has the same taste for all of us. I think the blues do too. Connecting with someone else who is struggling can help us realize that we're not alone. Reaching out to another person also takes us out of our self-focused thoughts. The impulse to turn our focus inward to our sick and pain-filled bodies can be a strong one. Indeed, it's understandable and, at times, skillful; we want to do everything we can to find the most beneficial treatments and maximize our functionality. That said, this tendency to turn inward can make us more susceptible to the blues.

Reaching out to others eases my blue mood. The gesture can take the simplest form: a short email to someone or a supportive comment on Facebook. It doesn't take much to brighten another person's day, and that sunlit brightness may kick up a breeze and blow those blues away.

There's no reason to be afraid of the blues. People in excellent health get them, so of course we do too. Our blues can be intense at times because they often center around the frustration and hopelessness we feel about our medical condition. But even if they're intense, they'll change—just like the weather.

It might help to keep these suggestions nearby because, if your life is like mine, the blues are never polite enough to announce ahead of time that they plan to spend the day.

15

Surviving a Bad Mood with Grace

Use your own problems to remember that others
have problems too.

—KATHLEEN MCDONALD

THANKFULLY, I don't get in bad moods very often, but when I do, it feels awful. Unlike when I have the blues, I don't feel melancholy. And I'm not on the verge of tears. Who can be bothered with tears? I'm too busy being cranky and irritable. I've isolated three types of bad moods, the last one exclusive to those with chronic illness.

The first type takes me by surprise; it shows up for no apparent reason. When it happens, I'm feeling fine one minute; then suddenly I'm in a bad mood, and every little thing annoys me. When a bad mood descends on me inexplicably in this way, I'm at such a loss to explain its cause that sometimes I think it must be due to something I ate!

The second type of bad mood comes on when a host of life's

little irritations adds up. A recent bad mood of my mine was set off in just this fashion. I misplaced a screw I needed to fix our doggy gate. I was having trouble untangling a cord to a bamboo shade. I couldn't figure out the instructions for programming a kitchen timer that my husband had recently bought. The final straw was the most innocuous (and perhaps common) of life's irritations: I could not find a sock in the dryer. All were minor irritations, yet they added up until there I was, in a bad mood. This particular bad mood was *so* bad that it qualified for what we (un)affectionately refer to in our household as a foul mood.

Finally, there's the bad mood that's unique to those with chronic illness. We can become weary that every day, year after year, we've been sick or we've been in pain... or both. Sometimes, the relentlessness of it all understandably triggers the irritation and crankiness of a bad mood.

This chapter offers some suggestions for surviving bad moods of all varieties.

Make an effort not to inflict the mood on others.

I try hard not to inflict a bad mood on those around me. When I slip up, I push myself to apologize even if I don't feel like it. Not only is an apology a nice gesture toward another, I've also noticed that it can lessen the intensity of a bad mood. I think it's because when we apologize, we're forced to reach out to another person and that takes us out of our self-focused mindset.

Don't be self-critical about the mood.

I've yet to spend time with anyone who hasn't been in a bad mood now and then. In a May 2010 interview with *Time* magazine, the Dalai Lama said that he still gets angry; I assume this means that he still can get in a bad mood. Many years ago, I had a Buddhist teacher who was wise and insightful... and subject to bad moods. I never knew what mood I'd encounter when I met with him.

If these two people can be in a bad mood, we should cut ourselves some slack when it happens to us. Why should being chronically ill make it inappropriate for us to ever be in a bad mood? That would be holding ourselves to a standard we'd never expect of others. Adding a negative judgment to a bad mood, such as "I shouldn't feel this way," serves only to increase the likelihood that the bad mood will turn into a foul one.

So instead of being self-critical when a bad mood hits, be okay with it—what's a little crankiness and irritability now and then? They're simply two among the seemingly infinite emotions that everyone experiences in life.

Investigate the mood.

Recall that in chapter 8, on patience, I set out a four-step approach for working mindfully with an unpleasant mood or emotion. The third step was to investigate it. Sometimes this can yield surprisingly fruitful results. A few years ago, in the days leading up to Christmas, I was in a bad mood. My husband seemed quite cheerful, so I resolved not to inflict it on him. Instead, I decided to investigate why I was in such a funk.

I know that I can be a bit sad during the holidays. Even so, I couldn't recall ever being this cranky and irritable, so I began to consciously think about my life at this time of year. Doing so, I uncovered a negative association I have with Christmas: I associate it with loss—one loss after another.

When I was ten years old, my father fell ill and then died just before Christmas. I felt his absence every Christmas after that until I met my husband and began to spend the holidays with his family. My father-in-law, Huey, took the place of my dad. They were both kind and good-natured men. I even remember telling my husband that his dad had become my Santa Claus because Huey embodied good will and the cheerful spirit of Christmas. Then Huey died when I was thirty-seven, and Christmas lost its luster again.

For several years, I took refuge in the traditions we developed with our children, Jamal and Mara. Then they grew up, had families of their own, and started their own holiday traditions. We know we're welcome to join them—Mara at her house in Los Angeles and Jamal at his in-laws near San Diego—but I'm too sick to travel. Another loss associated with Christmas.

This reflective investigation led me to see that the mild sadness I tend to feel when the holidays roll around had turned into a bad mood this year simply because of the cumulative effect of all those losses. As soon as I realized that I associate Christmas with loss, my bad mood turned into a sad mood—a familiar sadness that softened my heart and made it possible for compassion to arise over how hard this time of year can be for me. When I compassionately accepted those losses as part of my life story, the sadness slowly lifted, and I was able to make the best of the Christmas that lay before me.

A good way to investigate a bad mood when you know its source is to challenge the assumptions behind it. I recall a day, several years ago, when I was in a bad mood as a result of my mind churning with a list of grievances about being sick day in and day out. Inspired by Byron Katie, I decided to see what would happen if I turned my grievances around (a practice I described in chapter 13). I picked up a pen and told myself to list everything I liked about being sick.

I started this little exercise without much faith in its ability to improve my mood. However, by the time I put the pen down, I was surprised to find that forcing myself to think about what I liked about being sick had wiped out that bad mood altogether. Here are four of the twelve items that were on my list: I don't answer to an alarm clock; I'm never stuck in traffic; no more awkward cocktail party silences; my to-do list is very short.

Investigation is a valuable tool for uncovering what might lie behind a bad mood and for challenging any faulty assumptions we might be making about our lives.

Put the mood in perspective and consider reaching out to someone in need.

Thinking about how a bad mood seems minor when compared to the suffering in the world can put the mood into perspective, although I should be clear: the purpose of doing this is not to blame ourselves for being in a bad mood. As I pointed out earlier in the chapter, everyone is subject to them. So don't be hard on yourself; we're simply putting a bad mood into perspective to lessen its intensity.

What would it be like to be raising children in a war zone, never knowing when explosives may hit our houses? What is life like for refugees who live in tent cities because of civil unrest or natural disasters? Sometimes if I'm in a bad mood and see a news story about how others are forced to live, I turn to my husband and say, "I may be sick, but I am so lucky," and my bad mood subsides.

Putting a bad mood into perspective like this can also inspire us to reach out to someone in need. As Kathleen McDonald suggests in the epigraph that begins this chapter: "Use your own problems to remember that others have problems too." As is the case with the blues, turning our attention away from ourselves and reaching out to others is a skillful way to lessen the intensity of a painful mood.

I used to worry that a bad mood was the sign of a "new me"—that it was here to stay—but no bad mood has ever taken up permanent residence in my mind. This is because a mood is a mental state that arises due to the coming together of causes and conditions, and those causes and conditions change.

As with the blues, it's better not to try and force a bad mood to go away. That kind of command can set up a stubborn resistance in our minds, which invariably makes a bad mood worse. It's much more effective to disarm the mood by greeting it with friendliness, even though, like the blues, it's an uninvited guest.

Then, remembering the impermanent and fleeting nature of all our moods, we can simply let the bad mood be, while at the same time treating ourselves with compassion over how unpleasant crankiness and irritability feel. Knowing that a bad mood is only a temporary visitor helps us hold it more lightly. We can remind ourselves, "It's no big deal," and then patiently wait, without aversion, until it runs its course and passes out of the mind. While we're waiting, we might do something nice for ourselves, like cuddling a pet or making a favorite hot drink.

16

Shedding the Burden of Embarrassment

You are taught that there is something wrong with you and
that you are imperfect. But there isn't and you're not.

—CHERI HUBER

I SUSPECT THAT EVERYONE reading this knows what it's like
to feel embarrassed. Embarrassment is the awkward self-
consciousness that arises when we think we've said or done something that makes us look foolish in front of others. Although it
differs from shame in that shame can be experienced over something known only to ourselves, like shame, embarrassment carries
with it an element of self-blame. It's a painful emotion because,
when we're embarrassed, we feel intensely uncomfortable with
ourselves.

Embarrassment has two root causes, both of which may be the
result of conditioning from early childhood. The first is our tendency to set unrealistically high standards for ourselves and then
feel embarrassed when, inevitably, we can't meet them. The second
is our tendency to evaluate ourselves based on what we assume

other people are thinking about us. Even though those assumptions are often erroneous, we convince ourselves that we're not living up to others' expectations, and this leads us to feel embarrassed.

The Chrysalis Incident

Before I got sick, I could get embarrassed over the slightest misstep, no matter how innocent. One of the most embarrassing incidents of my life happened over thirty years ago. My husband was a graduate student, and we lived on an apricot ranch near the university. In the summer, I helped bring in much-needed income by working in the drying sheds. My job was to take an apricot out of a crate, cut it in half, expel the pit, and put the apricot on a drying tray. It took me over an hour to finish a crate and for that effort I earned two bucks.

One morning, in excitement, I shared with a coworker that I'd just found out I was pregnant. After our lunch break, she came up to me with something pretty in the palm of her hand and said, "This is to celebrate your pregnancy." Thinking it was a rock (she knew I collected them), I took it out of her palm without delicacy. Suddenly, it started oozing liquid on my fingers. She looked at me in horror and yelled, "What are you doing? That's a chrysalis!"

What I'd assumed to be a rock was actually the hard skin that covers a caterpillar as it is metamorphosing into a butterfly. If a chrysalis becomes detached from the silk pad that the caterpillar has spun but is handled very gently, it can be reattached and still become a butterfly. This one would not become a butterfly. I'd seen to that.

I was so embarrassed that I spent the rest of the day feeling painfully self-conscious. I wanted to be invisible. My embarrassment was made worse by my assumption that whenever my coworker was talking to others, she was telling them about what I'd done.

This is a classic illustration of the two reasons why people get embarrassed. First, I'd set an unrealistically high standard for myself. What crime had I committed by innocently mistaking a chrysalis for a rock? Are we to never misidentify an object? Second, I was evaluating myself based on what I assumed other people were thinking about me. This intensified my embarrassment and the self-blame I was directing at myself, even though I had no evidence to back up my assumption that my coworker was talking to others about what I had done.

For over thirty years, whenever I recalled that incident, I'd suffer embarrassment all over again. I use the word "suffer" on purpose because, for decades, conjuring up that memory made me miserable.

It can be eye-opening to become mindful of some of the unrealistic standards we hold ourselves to. These are the "shoulds" we set up in our lives—shoulds that become the breeding ground for embarrassment: I should never spill a drink; I should never lose my footing, even on slippery pavement; I should never misunderstand another person's behavior.

For most of my life, violating one of these self-selected "shoulds" has been a source of embarrassment, although the "chrysalis incident" was always the worst in my mind. If at the time I'd been able to feel compassion for myself instead of jumping straight to negative self-judgment, I could have said to my coworker something like "Oh, I'm terribly sorry. I thought it was a rock. I wish I'd have seen what it really was." Then the momentary discomfort would have passed without lingering in my mind for decades.

Chronic Illness and Embarrassment

Ironically, being chronically ill has helped me overcome my tendency to get embarrassed—ironic, because chronic illness tends to make people *more* embarrassment-prone. It's easy to see why. The unrealistically high standard at work here is that we don't think we *should* be chronically ill. Even though 130 million people suffer from chronic illness in the United States alone, we live in a culture that repeatedly suggests that, with proper diet and lifestyle changes, no one need be sick and no one need be in pain. When we're not living up to what we perceive to be that cultural standard, we feel embarrassed.

The first few years after I got sick, I was "chronically embarrassed" over not being able to recover my health. Other people get sick and recover. What was wrong with me that this wasn't happening? It didn't occur to me that I was holding myself to an unrealistic standard—unrealistic in the sense that I can't control whether my body recovers from a virus or not.

This embarrassment was fed by my ongoing worry over what other people might be thinking about me. After all, they're also products of this "everyone-can-be-healthy" culture. I was particularly concerned that they could be thinking I was a malingerer—someone who feigns illness in order to avoid work and other responsibilities. This led me to hide from others how sick I felt. If a colleague stopped me in the hallway of the law school during the short period of time that I continued to work, I'd lean against the wall as we chatted so he or she couldn't tell that I was barely able to stand up. I sat in the classroom to teach, so students wouldn't know that I was sick (although some of them figured it out). I did everything I could to hide my illness because it I felt so embarrassed by it.

Then I had a simple interaction with a neighbor that was a turning point in my life because it enabled me to begin to shed the terrible burden of embarrassment. I was in front of my house when a neighbor walked up and started chatting about the gardens on our block. After about ten minutes, I began to feel as if I would keel over if I couldn't find some support, but there was no wall to lean against as there'd been at the law school.

In the past, this would have been the trigger for embarrassment and self-blame to arise. Instead, there was a mental shift. I now think of it as a moment when I reached out to myself with compassion. Instead of trying to hide my illness, I said to my neighbor, "I'm sorry, but it's hard for me to stand up for long periods so I need to sit down." And because there was no chair in sight, I sat right down on the cement sidewalk! Sitting there, I continued our chat even though she towered over me. I wasn't embarrassed because I recognized that my intention was benevolent—to take care of myself.

Later, when I reflected on this interaction, I was astonished at what I'd done. I was a person who'd get embarrassed if I tripped on the sidewalk, but in that moment I'd been perfectly willing to sit right down on it. I reflected on what would happen if I stopped focusing on what other people might be thinking about me (which is more often than not an incorrect perception anyway). To help with this, I asked myself whether other people do the same things that I'd been judging myself so harshly for all my life. Do other people spill drinks? Yes. Do other people trip on sidewalks? Yes. Do other people misunderstand others sometimes? Yes. Do other people sometimes engage in unconventional behavior in order to protect their health? Yes!

This helped me put all those embarrassments into the larger context of what we as humans are likely to do and have happen to us. Then I purposefully called the "chrysalis incident" to mind. Might other people have mistaken that chrysalis for a rock? Yes. Might the very coworker who gave it to me have made that mistake? Of course.

Had I not become chronically ill, I might still be embarrassed about that chrysalis. Now, instead of embarrassment arising when I think of that day in the drying shed, I feel compassion for the excited young woman I was, who did nothing more than make an innocent mistake as she stood there ready to receive a gift to celebrate her pregnancy.

I hope that if you're feeling embarrassed about the state of your health, this chapter has helped you see that you need not hold yourself to the unrealistic standard of "I shall not be chronically ill." Bodies get sick, and they get injured and old. I also hope you won't set this standard: "I shall not engage in any unconventional behavior to accommodate my medical struggles." This idea is not only unrealistic; it lacks self-compassion.

Regardless of whether you make an innocent mistake (as I did with that chrysalis) or whether you behave unconventionally (as I did when I sat on the sidewalk), embarrassment serves no purpose. It's not compassionate because it doesn't ease your suffering—or anyone else's. And it doesn't promote equanimity. In fact, embarrassment and the peaceful abiding of equanimity seem to be opposites. Embarrassment is characterized by unease and discomfort because you think you should be other than what or who you are. By contrast, equanimity is characterized by a feeling of ease and comfort with yourself.

To find this place of ease and comfort, first acknowledge with kindness that sometimes you'll make innocent mistakes. Second, recognize that your behavior might not always meet others' expectations. Third, and most important for equanimity, vow to work on being okay with both of these inevitable life experiences.

IV. Special Challenges

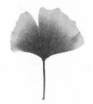

17

Invisibility: When You Look Fine to Others

It is only with one's heart that one can see clearly.
What is essential is invisible to the eye.

—ANTOINE DE SAINT-EXUPÉRY

ONE OF THE experiences that caught me by surprise when I got sick was the realization that I'd taken up residence in a parallel universe I hadn't even known existed: the invisible world of the chronically ill. The reason it's invisible is that most of us who live in it don't appear on the surface to be any different from those around us. Many of us simply don't look or sound as if we're sick or in pain.

Millions of people live day-to-day with medical problems that are invisible to others. This often includes conditions that are life threatening, such as cancer and heart disease. I read about a young man with primary sclerosing cholangitis, a serious autoimmune disorder of the liver. His situation was life-threatening—he was on a waiting list for a liver transplant—but on the outside he looked fine.

And I remember seeing tennis great Venus Williams on television shortly after she was diagnosed with Sjögren's syndrome, an autoimmune disease. The announcers were talking about her illness as the camera moved in for a close-up. As I watched, I was certain that most viewers would be thinking, "But she doesn't *look* sick." I've met a woman online who suffers from Sjögren's, so I knew that Williams was facing a hard struggle. I also knew that it was largely an invisible one.

There are consequences to having dual residences—in the world inhabited by the healthy as well as in the invisible world of the chronically ill. This chapter will explore them.

Guilt

Because we're repeatedly told that we look and sound fine, many of us feel guilty about being chronically ill. We've talked ourselves into believing that we must be doing something wrong because we're not "beating" it. As I've noted throughout the book, the culture we live in reinforces this notion. Yes, it's okay to occasionally come down with an acute illness or be in pain due to an injury or a surgical procedure, but then we're supposed to get better. Everyone expected it of me, and I expected it of myself.

For many years, I felt guilty that I wasn't living up to this cultural norm. I thought I was failing an obligation to others and to myself to get better. This emotional reaction can add intense mental suffering to the physical suffering that the chronically ill are already living with every day.

The cultural message that everybody has the ability to be in good health is especially hard on young people because they face additional pressure to "hit the gym" and stay in shape. Until I became a member of the chronic illness community, I didn't realize how many young people struggle with their health. In chapter 19, I discuss the extra difficulties they face.

These feelings of guilt may extend to those we're closest to. In the early years of my illness, I used to sob to my husband, "I've ruined your life." I count myself fortunate to have had his shoulder to cry on; many spouses and partners don't stick around, leaving the chronically ill person alone, sometimes to raise the couple's children. Many chronically ill parents have written to me about the terrible guilt they feel over their inability to be the active parent they'd always dreamed they'd be.

I understand what they're going through because I had to overcome the painful guilt I felt over not being active in the lives of my two grandchildren. I had so many fantasies about what we'd be doing together. My oldest grandchild Malia lives in the city where I grew up—Los Angeles. I thought I'd be taking her to all my favorite places. My youngest grandchild Cam lives in Berkeley, only about an hour from where I live. I thought I'd be riding cable cars with her in San Francisco and taking her on bay cruises that would go right under the Golden Gate Bridge. Instead, I seldom leave the house.

It was only when I applied my mindfulness skills that I realized it wasn't my fault that I was sick. The Buddha's teachings were immensely helpful to me here. He offers that dose of realism I've referred to before: this is what it means to be born into a body. It's part of the human experience that bodies get sick and injured and old. Once I accepted this, I was able to shed the guilty feeling that I was letting my grandchildren—and everyone else—down. Then I could embrace my life as it is—sickness included. This freed me to look for ways to connect with my grandchildren that didn't include seeing them in person very often, such as Skyping and texting. I particularly love texting because it doesn't matter how I look!

Embarrassment

Influenced by cultural norms, many of us worry that others are judging us negatively because of our health problems. As discussed in the previous chapter, this can be the source of painful embarrassment. And if our chronic condition happens to be invisible, that embarrassment can increase twofold.

It did for me in the early years of my illness. Because I didn't look sick or in pain, I dreaded running into people I knew. I assumed that when they saw how normal I looked, they'd judge me negatively for not being an active member of the workforce or the community anymore. My embarrassment could be so intense that I often wished I looked as terrible as I felt.

Invisible illness can be a particular source of embarrassment for parents with school-aged children. Several of them have written to me about how embarrassed they feel when they have to decline requests from other parents or school officials to take a more active role in their children's activities, such as chaperoning field trips. These parents are convinced that those around them think they're simply trying to avoid doing their fair share.

A good antidote for embarrassment is to remind ourselves that our perceptions about others can be wrong. There's no reason to assume that just because we don't look sick or in pain, everyone we interact with will judge us negatively if we share that we're chronically ill. In the same way that we hope other people will give us the benefit of the doubt, we'd do well to initially give it to them.

Fear of Being Misunderstood

The list of misunderstandings about chronic illness is a long one; I write about some of them in chapter 34, "Setting the Record Straight about Chronic Illness." Here are three more.

Because our condition is invisible, we may be treated as lazy or as malingerers by family members, friends, employers, the medical profession, even the general public. After I was interviewed on a local National Public Radio show, I received an email from a listener telling me that he didn't want his tax dollars going to support "an amotivational slacker." At the time I read the email, it stung—badly. I was helped by my friend Jane; when I shared his words with her, she pointed out how unhappy he must be to have said something so cruel to me. Her response—compassion for him—dissipated the painful anger that I was directing at him.

Second, due to the lack of visible cues about our chronic illness, we are often misunderstood by the medical community. Some doctors look at us and, seeing that we look fine, prescribe strenuous exercise—the very activity that is likely to exacerbate our symptoms. Or we may be labeled as "drug seekers" in emergency rooms and, as a result, be denied necessary pain medication. Several people have told me that, unless their personal doctor is available to vouch for them, they won't go to the emergency room, no matter how unbearable their pain becomes.

Lastly, we face misunderstanding about what it means to be disabled. Just because we're too sick to work and be active for extended periods doesn't mean we can't sometimes do things around the house or have friends over.

Sometimes I don't tell others that I'm planning to do something that healthy people do—such as going out to dinner. I've learned that other chronically ill people do the same thing. Why would we deliberately hide our plans to do something special? Because from years of living in the parallel universe of the chronically ill, we've learned that when people see us out and about, they're likely to assume that our health has improved. Then we have to field well-meaning—but off-base—comments, such as "I'm so glad you're feeling well enough to go out." We're not feeling well enough. We're just doing it anyway.

Hiding plans like this does not feel good to me, especially because it includes not sharing my experience with people afterward. This, of course, increases my sense of isolation from others. To share or not to share is a balancing act that the chronically ill are continually engaged in. I'm aware that sometimes I let the scales tip in the wrong direction.

Misunderstanding what it means to be disabled can have tragic consequences. I've read about people who've had their long-term disability payments revoked because an investigator who was sent to check up on them saw them being active in some way. In one such instance, a woman lost her disability check after the investigator saw her doing light gardening in her front yard. That's sobering: as limited as I am, I sometimes pull weeds; I can't ask my husband to do *everything*.

These are some of the challenges faced by those of us whose medical conditions are invisible. It can feel as if we're inhabiting two worlds—the one we share with the healthy and the invisible one we share with others who are chronically ill. Juggling these two worlds is a lot of work. As I've noted before, it's no wonder we sometimes feel that being chronically ill is a full-time job—a job we didn't train for and one we are often ill-equipped to perform.

Challenging though it may be, the burden falls on us to make the *invisible* visible to others. It's yet another part of our "workload." This entails educating people about chronic illness, something I discussed in detail in chapter 1.

What I say in that chapter applies here too: some people may never accept that we're disabled by an invisible chronic illness. That inability on their part is about them, not us. They may not have had previous experience with people who are sick or in pain.

It may scare them and remind them of their own mortality. In addition, they may never have learned how to be compassionate toward others. The kindest thing we can do for ourselves when this happens is to accept that disappointments like this are an inevitable part of life and then wrap ourselves in a cloak of self-compassion over any suffering we're experiencing as a result of their lack of understanding.

In those moments when I accept that some of the people I know may never understand what life with chronic illness is like for me, I'm able to let go of the painful longing and fruitless desire for them to behave as I want them to. It's like putting down a heavy load because I'm finally giving up a fight I cannot win. This gives rise to equanimity—that calm sense of peace and well-being with my life as it is, whether others understand it or not.

18

When You and Those You Love
Are in Conflict

Attention is the rarest and purest form of generosity.
—SIMONE WEIL

CHRONIC ILLNESS is one of life's most stressful experiences, so it's not surprising that it can put a strain on the closest relationships—romantic partners, family members, even best friends. As noted at the end of chapter 1, some of our loved ones may be unable to give us the kind of support we'd like to have, and it's essential to our peace of mind to work on accepting this with grace. Even with these people, however, it's possible to resolve conflicts that arise in our day-to-day life together. This chapter offers several techniques for doing this.

Initially, it may seem unfair that we who are coping every day with chronic illness have to take the lead in resolving conflicts with loved ones. If we look at the relationship from a different perspective, however, we'll realize that the people to whom we're closest are suffering right along with us. In my view, my husband has suffered as much as I have as a result of my illness and how it's turned upside down the life we expected to be sharing.

I think he'd disagree, saying that he doesn't have to live day in and day out with a body that's sick. And yet I've watched how hard it is for him. In addition to his ongoing worry about my health, he's taken on many extra responsibilities—and lost his partner out in the world. To me, he and I are in the same boat, and so if a conflict arises, I see no reason why I shouldn't be the one to try and help our relationship be as good as it can be.

Before reading these suggestions, you might think of a sensitive subject or current conflict that you'd like to raise with a loved one, whether that loved one is a partner, a family member, or a close friend.

Stick to the issue at hand.

A discussion about a conflict often starts out well, focusing on the issue at hand, but there's a tendency to drift. Suddenly, the discussion is about all the grievances in the relationship. When this happens, nothing is likely to be resolved.

Using mindfulness skills can help you keep the discussion on track. First, be sure it's clear in your mind exactly what the issue is. Then, before starting to speak, take a conscious breath or two to calm yourself and gather your thoughts. When you're ready, communicate to your loved one the *one thing* you'd like to work on resolving. For example, you might say: "I know we have several conflicts we could discuss, but can we focus on solving our disagreement about how to put the children to bed at night?"

At any point that the discussion drifts off-topic, take the initiative and return to the conflict you're trying to resolve. Focusing on one issue at a time increases the likelihood of coming to an agreement that's satisfactory to both of you.

Talk about how you feel, as opposed to what you think your loved one should be doing or not doing.

This suggestion comes from a technique I learned many years ago in one of my child-raising books. It's called sending "I-messages" instead of "You-messages." The idea is to try and avoid the use of the word "you," which makes the other person feel as if he or she is being accused of something. So instead of using phrases such as "you should" or "you shouldn't," stick to talking about your own feelings.

As an example, if a loved one doesn't do something he promised to do, instead of saying "You didn't do what you said you'd do" or the even more confrontational "You never do what you say you'll do," say something like "I feel frustrated." Expressing how *you* feel is much less likely to turn a disagreement into an argument because you're not blaming your loved one. You're simply explaining how you feel at the moment. In addition, it's easier to hold your ground; you feel the way you feel. No one can deny that.

Here are two more examples of how using "I-messages" can help resolve conflicts.

1. *The conflict*: Whenever you ask a loved one for help around the house, he or she gets upset, and you wind up in an argument. The other person could be your partner, a child, or a sibling.

   In this situation, when talking to your loved one, instead of saying "You should help more" or "You shouldn't get mad just because I ask for help," focus on your feelings by sending an "I-message." Try saying something like this: "I'm worried because I'm unable to handle all the household tasks. Could we make a list of things that need to be done and then divide them up in a way that looks manageable for both of us? We can revisit the list in a few days to see if it needs adjusting."

2. *The conflict*: When you're in bad pain, your loved one ignores you, as if it can't possibly be that bad.

In raising this, instead of sending a "You-message," such as "You should believe me when I say I'm in pain" or "You shouldn't ignore me when I'm in pain," focus on how it feels for you to have your pain disregarded. Try saying something like this: "On days when I'm in terrible pain, I feel bad that I don't know how to let you know how much I'm hurting. Can we discuss how I can talk to you about my pain levels in a way that would feel comfortable to you?"

Learning to speak this way takes practice, and it may feel awkward at first. Most of us are in the habit of communicating by using "You-messages." I certainly am. In addition, an "I-message" can inadvertently or intentionally be a disguised "You-message." In the above example about pain levels, if you'd said, "I feel bad that you refuse to acknowledge my pain," your comment would have started out as an "I-message" but quickly turned into a "You-message."

If you try the technique and don't get the wording right, it's okay. From the heart, say, "I'm sorry": "I'm sorry. Can I take back what I said and try to say it in a clearer and more helpful way?"

Put yourself in your loved one's shoes.

Putting yourself in the other person's shoes helps resolve conflicts because it breaks you free from the stubbornly held position that the only solution is for your loved one to see things your way. When your mind gets stuck in "my way is the only right way," conflict resolution becomes virtually impossible, partly because that mindset often gives rise to anger. In fact, "I'm right and you're wrong" is a common theme underlying anger.

Understanding a conflict from the other person's point of view helps you see that a seemingly callous or indifferent reaction to the difficulties in your relationship does not automatically mean that your loved one doesn't care about you. Instead, it may reflect his or her worries and fears about your medical condition—a reaction that stems from love and concern for you. Understanding this makes it easier not to take your loved one's behavior personally.

The best way to see the conflict from your loved one's point of view is to engage in "active listening" (also called "empathetic listening"). This is a technique I learned when my two children were young. Even though I wasn't always as skillful at it as I wanted to be, it was extremely helpful to them at times. The goal is to let the other person know that you've truly heard his or her concerns. To do this, you feed back to your loved one, in your own words, what you think he or she is feeling.

For example, if your daughter is afraid of the dark, instead of trying to talk her out of how she's feeling by saying "There's no reason to be afraid of the dark" or "You're too old to be afraid of the dark," you feed back her feelings to her by saying "The dark is scary to you." When you actively listen in this way, your daughter feels heard and validated. This makes it easier for her to overcome a fear because she knows you're taking her concern seriously, and she knows that you're trying to understand it from her point of view.

This technique is equally effective in the context of chronic illness. It's not uncommon for family members to be struggling with the upheaval in both of your lives, not to mention worries over issues that may have become more pressing and serious as a result of your illness, such as finances, isolation, and what the future holds.

For example, perhaps you want your partner to accompany you to doctor appointments, partly for support and partly so that he or she can learn more about your medical condition and the challenges you face. If your partner refuses to go, your first reaction might be to assume that he or she doesn't care enough about you to be bothered. And yet the very opposite might be true: your partner may love you so much that it's too hard to be a witness to your suffering.

To actively listen in this situation, you demonstrate to your partner that you understand how he or she feels by putting those feelings into your own words: "I understand why you might prefer not to come with me to the doctor. You're so busy with other things, and it's not a particularly pleasant experience for you anyway. I think that if you came, though, we'd both have a better idea of what's going on with my health. Then we could work on making life as easy and pleasant as possible for both of us. What do you think?" Then listen carefully to what he or she says.

When you actively listen in this way, loved ones feel heard and validated; they see that you're not challenging their point of view. Instead, you're making an effort to understand it. This makes it more likely that you can talk openly together about the conflict at hand.

In those moments when I'm able to put myself in my loved ones' shoes and see my illness through their eyes, compassion arises for them. If this happens to you and makes you want to reach out—do. A hand on a hand, a rub across the back, a hug can do wonders to alleviate tension when two people are in a conflict. The slightest show of affection can break a deadlock, and then you can begin anew. Every moment is a chance to begin anew. Often both people in a conflict want this to happen, but no one wants to be the first person to reach out. If you can, *be* that person.

Know thyself... and then try something different.

When raising sensitive subjects with a loved one, you can communicate more effectively if you know your own tendencies when you're in a conflict situation. Are you quick to get angry? Do you start yelling, or do you withdraw and become very quiet? Do you get sarcastic? Are you "the nice one" who always wants to accommodate others in any way possible because you don't like conflict or are afraid of it?

Set an intention to become mindful of how you respond when you're in a conflict with someone. It might not be obvious to you at first, so take some time and see if you can pinpoint your behavior.

You can use this bit of self-knowledge to help break down communication deadlocks that tend to arise when the subject you've raised is a sensitive one. By switching your usual mode of behaving, you can avoid the established ruts of your relationship. And when your loved one witnesses this unfamiliar behavior from you, he or she is more likely to pay careful attention to what you're saying. So if you tend to withdraw, instead speak up. If you tend to get angry, instead resolve to stay calm. I'll share my experience with this technique so you can see why I recommend it.

The more upset I get about something, the more I tend to lower my voice and speak quietly. I didn't realize this until a friend pointed it out to me years ago as she watched me handle a conflict with my toddler son. When I do this, I appear calm on the outside, but it's a fake calm; inside, I'm tense and upset.

When I read about this tactic of switching your behavior, I decided to give it a try. The next time I found myself in a conflict with a loved one, I made a conscious effort to speak up. I didn't start yelling—that's rarely a good way to communicate—but I raised the volume of my voice. I was so astonished to hear myself speaking up in this way that I found myself being much more articulate in communicating my concerns about the conflict at hand.

In addition, I noticed that my loved one was taken aback. He sat up a bit straighter and paid more attention to what I had to say. The conversation that followed was constructive and productive; to my surprise, we resolved the problem quite easily.

Look upon compromise as a positive outcome.

Don't go into a discussion of a conflict with the attitude that one of you will "win" and one of you will "lose." Not only is this likely to leave bad feelings, but it's not necessary for resolving most conflicts.

To illustrate this point, let's go back to one of the conflicts I mentioned: putting the children to bed at night. A good way to resolve the conflict might be for each of you to give in a bit on what you think is ideal. If you're disagreeing over the time to set for their bedtime, you could agree to compromise. Or you could compromise over the bedtime ritual, such as how many books you'll read to them.

Compromise might also be an effective way to resolve the conflict over wanting a partner to accompany you to a doctor's appointment. You could agree that he or she will come every other time or whenever you indicate that something important will be discussed at the appointment.

If you can resolve a conflict by each of you giving in a bit or by coming up with a new alternative that meets both of your needs, then you've done more than just resolve the issue—both of you have come away from the discussion feeling respected by the other. This is good for the overall health of your relationship. To quote the Vietnamese Zen monk and teacher Thich Nhat Hanh: "In true dialogue, both sides are willing to change."

The stresses that chronic illness can bring to close relationships makes the challenge of finding peace with your new life even more difficult. Although the techniques in this chapter take practice, in my experience, they're worth the effort. I'm not suggesting that they'll magically resolve all the conflicts you have with those you love. And if you've reached an impasse over a serious conflict, you might consider professional counseling; the presence of a neutral third party in the room can facilitate more calm and constructive communication.

It's also okay for some conflicts to remain unresolved. Close relationships can thrive even when there are disagreements, so long as each of you respects the other's point of view. The best way to be sure you're doing that is to practice being mindful of how each conflict appears in the eyes of your loved one.

19

The Special Difficulties Faced by Young People Who Are Chronically Ill

It takes courage to grow up and become who you really are.

—E. E. CUMMINGS

BEFORE I BECAME a member of the community of the chronically ill, I thought that young people—at least through their thirties—were either healthy (aside from the occasional cold or flu) *or* had a terminal illness. I had no idea that millions of young people live day-to-day with chronic illness. They suffer from symptoms that, while not necessarily life-threatening, affect every aspect of their lives: unrelenting pain, debilitating fatigue, shortness of breath or vertigo, damage to vital organs such as the lungs and kidneys. Many of them have spent a good part of their childhood and young adulthood in medical settings; some have undergone multiple surgeries.

This chapter focuses on the difficulties faced by young people with chronic illness, although much of it can apply to people of any age.

Being treated as if your medical problem can't possibly be chronic.
In this culture, the words "young" and "acute illness" appear to go
together, but "young" and "chronic illness" do not. Young people tell me that family and friends often treat them as if they can't
possibly have a medical condition that might last a lifetime. This
leaves them feeling frustrated, hurt, and sad.

When young people are disregarded in this way, they may even
begin to question their own perceptions: "Am I really in pain all
the time? Everyone says it can't possibly be the case, so maybe it's
all in my head." This self-doubt can lead to self-recrimination and
can seriously erode a young person's sense of self-worth. Many
of them have told me that the greatest gift a loved one could give
them would be to say, "I believe you."

In addition, young people face discrimination by the population
as a whole, especially if their illness is invisible—as is often the
case. Several young people have told me that they've been openly
challenged when they park in a disabled spot, even though they
have the required placard or sticker. (By contrast, no one has ever
challenged me.)

If a stranger is rude to you in this fashion, the best response is
to acknowledge to yourself that you feel hurt, take a deep breath,
and then immediately turn your attention to taking loving care of
yourself. Don't let another person's insensitivity make you question yourself. The problem lies with that person's ignorance about
chronic illness; it does not lie with you. Make a commitment to
become your own unconditional ally. This is the essence of self-
compassion. With practice, it can become a lifelong habit. Start by
separating this person's behavior from what you know to be true
about yourself. In other words, *you know you're sick; you know
you're in pain*. Let that be good enough for you.

It saddens me every time I hear about a young person who is
chronically ill being challenged by other people. Everyone should

be given the benefit of the doubt. No one is too young to suffer from chronic illness.

Being repeatedly told, "You're too young to be in pain."

I'm not young, so no one has said this to me. However, I've lost count of the number of young people who've written to me, saying that this is one of the most frustrating comments they have to listen to. Sometimes they're even told they're too young to have the very illness they've been diagnosed with, especially if it's something that's associated with being older, such as osteoarthritis. Then they have to listen to remarks like "No one your age gets arthritis" or "You're too young to be in pain from arthritis." These types of comments are a challenge for young people to respond to skillfully because they're being told that they're not experiencing what they are, in fact, experiencing.

Perhaps most destructive to a young person is being told by a doctor that he or she can't possibly be seriously ill or in pain. At the end of one of my online articles, a young woman described having had this experience:

> I'm only twenty-two and I had to literally beg my doctor to let me get an MRI. She kept telling me no because I was too young to have anything seriously wrong. She finally let me get one and we found out that I have juvenile degenerative disc disease and quite a few herniated discs. By the time I had my surgery, my surgeon said he couldn't believe that I was able to wait as long as I did because it was so bad and I must have been in so much pain. I've already had one back surgery and I'm probably headed for a second one soon.

If you're young and have been told by a doctor that your condition can't possibly be chronic or that you're too young to be in pain, do your best to find another doctor. If you're being told this by family and friends, it's good to remember that you might not be able to change their minds. It makes sense to try and educate them, but keep in mind that a recurring theme in this book is that not everyone comes through for us. When you feel disappointed by others, try thinking about it this way: it's better to have two friends and family members who believe you and are interested in what life is like for you than to have a dozen who don't.

Many of my friends dropped away when I became chronically ill. I've learned to treasure the few who've stuck around and the few who've newly entered my life, because I know they don't question the chronic nature of my illness. I've learned to let the others go. This is an equanimity practice: working on accepting that people's behavior will not always conform to your wishes and being content with those who are there to support you.

Being isolated from others your age.

My heart ached for the mother of a chronically ill young woman as I read this comment she posted at the end of one of my online articles:

> The alienation of friends has been very painful for my daughter. She feels so alone and I don't know how to fix this problem. If something happens to me, she has no one and I worry every night. I wish her friends would be true friends and comfort her and spend time with her.

Being isolated from peers can be one of the most traumatic consequences of chronic illness in the young. The ability to interact with others their age offers welcome relief from the constant focus on their heath, even if it's just chatting about a favorite reality TV show. In addition, hanging out with peers—comparing interests, discussing likes and dislikes—helps young people form their identity and prepares them to blossom as adults. If you're young, I hope you'll keep reaching out to others—in person or online. There may be some disappointments in store for you when you do this, but one good friend can make a world of difference in your life.

Having to watch other young people engage in activities that are out of reach.

A few years ago, I read an article in *The Atlantic* that was written by the wife of a thirty-three-year-old man who'd been diagnosed with the autoimmune disease ankylosing spondylitis, which causes inflammation of the spinal vertebrae. In the article, she quoted her husband describing how difficult and polarizing it was to be with people who weren't sick:

> It's, like, I'm still only thirty-three. I probably am still considered in a lot of people's eyes youthful enough that I shouldn't have to deal with thinking about this kind of stuff. I feel like my parents were still partying and drinking beers [at 33]. This is the age my Dad was when they had me. I don't think [he] was worrying about what [expletive deleted] pills he was going to take or not take, you know what I mean? They were like, "We're out of Budweiser."

Many young people have had to give up active lifestyles as musicians, marathon runners, social activists, yoga instructors. They're frustrated and sometimes they're angry. Always, they're sad. Worst of all, they tend to blame themselves for their inability to be active. I tell them over and over that it's not their fault. I also encourage them to focus on what they *can* do and to look for others (online or in-person) who have similar interests.

Thinking outside the box can help. There may be activities you never considered before: macro-photography, where you need not leave your own backyard; joining an online arts or craft group, where you can learn from others and post pictures of your work; helping others from your phone or from the internet. If someone had told me I was going to become a writer from my bed, I would have said, "You're kidding, right?" Yet here I am, about to have my third book published. If you like to write and can't find a publisher, self-publish! Make "think outside the box" your mantra. The internet can be a great resource here.

Finding it impossible to complete college.

Higher education is generally a ticket to brighter employment prospects. But when chronic illness strikes, young people are often forced to drop out of school. I've received dozens of emails about this. Here are two samples: "I was unable to get my BA because of the unpredictability of whether I'd be able to attend classes on any given day"; "I was two-thirds of the way to my PhD when crippling pain forced me to drop out of the program."

In addition, many students must work part-time to help defray the costs of a college education. Young people who are chronically ill may not be able to do this. They already have two "jobs": the job of being a student and the job of taking care of their health. Even if they're able to keep up with their classes, they may not be able to add part-time work to their lives. This circumstance in itself can force young people to drop out of school.

When it comes to higher education, if you're young and chronically ill, once again, think outside the box. Treat this contemplation as part of the workload of that job of taking care of your health. Maybe you can find a dean of students or a counselor at your campus's disability services office who is willing to brainstorm with you to come up with some viable alternatives, such as moving to an extended program or taking some classes online.

When I served as the dean of students at the law school at UC Davis, I tried to help a young man who'd been sick with what the doctors initially thought was an acute viral infection. When, after six months, he still hadn't recovered, he was given the diagnosis of chronic fatigue syndrome. He was a dedicated student and was determined to get his law degree. When he and I realized that he could no longer keep up in his classes, I put him on a four-year program, which extended his studies by a year so that he could take a lighter class load. We thought this would allow him to complete his law degree.

Soon, however, he lost the ability to take care of his daily needs. Some days he couldn't get out of bed at all. As a result, in addition to having to miss classes, he could no longer get to the grocery store to buy food. It became increasingly clear that he could no longer live independently. And so, after completing three-fourths of the units toward his law degree, he had no choice but to withdraw from school and move back in with his parents, who lived in another state.

I felt so bad for him. Little did I know that eight years later, I'd be given the same diagnosis and be forced, in effect, to withdraw from the very same school.

Having trouble finding work and dealing with the financial fallout.

Young people who are chronically ill worry about their ability to compete in the job market with those who are healthy. There are federal and state antidiscrimination laws to protect those with disabilities, but there are subtle ways for employers to skirt those laws when deciding whom to hire from a large applicant pool.

Accompanying this obstacle is an ongoing concern about

finances. Even young people with good health insurance have to shoulder the costs of copays. And many nontraditional treatments that provide symptom relief, such as acupuncture, aren't covered by insurance. Having to allocate so much money for medical expenses can diminish a young person's quality of life. As one young woman told me: "Even when my chronic condition is under control, the debt from it is always there."

Being stigmatized by others.

Think about the burden that a chronically ill child must bear. When I was in elementary school, I got upset if I had a cold and had to miss a field trip. Imagine having to miss weeks of school at a time and not being able to participate in extracurricular activities. Additionally, such children may be stigmatized by others and suffer from terrible embarrassment.

When I was in grade school, all I wanted was to fit in—at least, not be noticed. There was a boy named Alan in my sixth grade class who suffered from asthma so severe that he missed weeks of school at a time. When he did show up, everyone knew "this is the kid who's always sick," and we treated him differently because of it. There was certainly no fitting in, no anonymity for Alan. He was stigmatized.

I realize now how terribly hard this must have been for him. He had to deal with both his illness and with his peers treating him as different. I hope he's had a good life, filled with love and understanding from family and friends. I wish I'd been compassionate enough to have been one of those friends.

Facing the possibility of not finding a romantic partner.

Living day-to-day with a limiting, unpredictable medical condition makes it hard to sustain any friendship, no matter how old you are. It's even harder to find romance. This can be an ongoing source of stress for young people who are chronically ill. They often have to severely limit how often and for how long they can be out and about, and this affects their ability to meet potential partners.

If they do meet someone, the relationship may stall in its tracks. A young woman with lupus recently wrote to me about a dinner date she'd had. The evening was going well, but when her date found out that she wouldn't be able to go to a concert on the weekend because she was scheduled to get chemotherapy, he lost interest in her altogether.

When I got sick, I was fortunate to have a committed partner who took our "in sickness and in health" vows seriously. When I reflect on my limitations, it's hard for me to imagine that I'd be able to find romance if I were young. It's a sobering thought. I may not get regular treatments, as does the young woman with lupus, but my illness severely restricts my ability to engage in activities. For example, if I wanted to go to a concert, the show would have to be during the day, be close to home, and last no more than two hours. What are the odds of that being the case?

And those criteria don't cover everything that would factor into whether I'd be able to attend or not. My symptoms are so unpredictable that, even if I agreed to go to the concert, when its scheduled date came around, I might be too sick to go. Cancelling plans at the last minute (especially plans that involve expensive tickets) is not conducive to beginning a romantic relationship.

On a positive note, romance can blossom if an understanding and patient person comes along. If you're young and chronically ill, try to think of creative ways to meet people. One woman told me that she met her fiancé online through a dating site. She said that the two of them had become so close as a result of their back and forth emails that, when they finally met in person, it mattered not a bit to him that she was disabled.

I used to be skeptical of online dating sites, but I know four perfectly matched couples who met this way. They're people about whom you'd say they wouldn't need the internet to help them find a partner. These sites turn out to be a very efficient way of finding people who share your interests, your values, and your life circumstances, including having to live with chronic illness. They're worth considering.

Deciding whether to have children.

A young woman in her middle thirties wrote to me saying that she'd been chronically ill for ten years. She was facing the question of whether or not to have children and wanted to get my opinion. She wasn't the first person to ask me about this. I'm not comfortable advising young people on these matters; so much depends on the nature of their illness and what kind of support system they have in place. Nevertheless, my heart aches whenever I get asked, because this is a question I never had to face. Well, almost never.

When I was twenty-five and pregnant with my son, I developed severe back pain. It was so debilitating that it became a major factor to consider when my husband and I decided to have a second child. In the end, we adopted a three-year-old girl from Korea. Now I cannot imagine any other child as my daughter. I raise this to focus, again, on the value of thinking outside the box and being willing to come up with creative solutions to whatever dilemma you're facing.

If caring for a child is more than you can handle, maybe you can be a second mother to one of your siblings' children. I've met two chronically ill women who've done just this. When I was a young child, my aunt's daughters were already grown and so she became an active part of my life, taking me on outings, lending a compassionate ear to my teenage problems. It became one of the most important relationships of my life.

Being worried and scared about the future.

People of all ages and health statuses worry about the future occasionally. But young people who are chronically ill have a lifetime of health-related worries ahead of them, worries that can escalate into fear: What will happen to my health in the years to come? Will my condition gradually worsen? Will I become more and more restricted in my activities? Will I be able to support myself? Will I be able to live independently, or will I become increasingly dependent on my family?

If you're young and chronically ill, I encourage you to talk with your family, friends, doctors, even a trusted counselor, such as a teacher, about these issues. The more information you can gather and the more support you have, the better equipped you'll be to plan for the future.

Being young and chronically ill is hard enough without taking into consideration the difficulties raised in this chapter. My heart goes out to these young people and their families, especially their parents who often become their caregivers. I've raised two children. I know how uneasy I felt every time one of them had an acute illness. I can only imagine how hard it would have been had one of them been chronically ill.

20

Maximizing Your Chances of Success at the Doctor's Office

You may not control all the events that happen to you,
but you can decide not to be reduced by them.
—MAYA ANGELOU

I'VE HAD my share of unsuccessful experiences with doctors, including being intimidated by them. Yes, this former law professor can allow herself to get intimidated by doctors! Finally, after many years of being chronically ill, I'm happy to report that I'm doing better in this uncomfortable setting, mainly because I've developed several strategies to help maximize my chances of success at the doctor's office.

**Think of the doctors and the staff as working for you,
not vice versa.**

I'm aware that this is an oversimplification of the legal relationships involved here, and I'm not suggesting that you order the doctors and the staff to do whatever you want. That said, I find it helpful to remind myself that they work for me in the same sense that an attorney or an accountant or a hairdresser does. I'm paying them for their expertise and their skill, even if the money goes through my insurance company. They are here to serve me, not vice versa.

Due to a combination of factors, it can be a challenge to maintain this perspective. First, you're in their territory—it's their turf. Second, it can feel as if they have all the knowledge and all the power, even though you may know more about your medical condition than they do. Third, you have to put on that nightgown-looking thingy that makes you look like a child. Fourth, you may be at your weakest in the doctor's office because the trip to get there, followed by the typical waiting times—first in the waiting room and then in the examination room—can take its toll even if you're having a relatively good day.

With my illness, I have to add to these four the fact that sometimes I'm too sick to sit in the examining room chair while waiting for the doctor so, as soon my vital signs have been taken, I lie down on the examining table to wait. When the doctor enters the room while I'm in this position—with that silly gown on—it's hard to feel as if this person who is towering over me works for me!

To help me remember who works for whom, as I sit (or lie) waiting, I often repeat to myself: "He works for me" or "She works for me." I also practice mindfulness by paying attention to what's present in my environment—the sights, the sounds, the smells. Doing this keeps me from focusing on any anxiety I'm experiencing about the upcoming interaction. After all, I can't be paying attention to what's presenting itself to my senses and, at the same time, be worrying about the future. If my mind wanders from the present moment to stressful thoughts about the appointment, as soon as I become aware this has happened, I repeat "He works for me" or "She works for me," and then return to bringing all my senses to bear on what's going on around me.

Consider taking someone with you.

Before I got sick in 2001, I had no idea that my husband could accompany me into the examining room. Now he comes with me whenever possible. No one has ever questioned his presence.

Having him there is beneficial for several reasons. First, I feel less intimidated when I know I have an ally with me who can vouch first-hand for how sick I am. Second, I've noticed that when doctors see him, they become more attentive to what I'm saying and are also more forthcoming with information and explanations. Doctors will often look over at my husband as if they're talking for his benefit. Sometimes when this happens, I feel like protesting, "Hey. Over here. I'm the patient. Talk to me!" but I refrain, because I'll take a more communicative doctor any way I can.

Third, if I'm having a tough day—a day when it's a major accomplishment just to have dragged myself to the appointment— he can be my advocate. He can raise new concerns or changes in my symptoms that I forget to mention; he can ask questions that may not have occurred to me. When he's there, I feel protected.

Fourth, on the way home, I get a second opinion about how the appointment went: Was the doctor a good listener? Did he or she involve me in the decision-making? Was the doctor open to treating a "no-quick-fix" patient?

Finally, if the appointment didn't go well, my husband can confirm my perception that I received less-than caring or competent treatment. This validation allows me to stop second-guessing myself. Even more, it gives rise to self-compassion because, with my husband's help, I'm able to see that this disappointing interaction with the doctor was not my fault.

You need not take a spouse or a partner. You can take anyone whom you feel comfortable with—an adult child or a cousin or a friend. If accompanying you to the doctor is a source of conflict between you and a loved one, look again at chapter 18 where I give an example of how you could approach this very issue.

Before you go to the appointment, tell the person who's coming with you what you're hoping to get out of the appointment and what you'd like him or her to be looking out for on your behalf. An extra pair or ears and eyes—and an extra brain—has been invaluable in helping me not to feel intimidated by even the most curt and brusque of doctors.

Recall from my story in chapter 4 about how I was unable to say no to the podiatrist who wanted to give me a second cortisone shot. I'm positive that had my husband been able to accompany me to that appointment, I'd have had the presence of mind to decline that shot.

Bring a list to the appointment.

Seven minutes is the average amount of time you get with the doctor under managed care. Thankfully, my primary care physician gives me more time than this, but I've encountered other doctors who are clearly working "on the clock." You can sense it when they walk into the room. In my experience, the best way to manage this is to bring a list of what you want to raise and have it visible to the doctor when he or she enters the room.

I make a list of what I want to talk about and then prioritize it. The list serves several purposes. First, it helps me manage my own time so I don't linger on one item too long, or stray off onto something I'd already decided wasn't important enough to raise at this appointment. (As my family well knows, I can easily go off topic!)

Second, when doctors see my list, they often prompt me by saying, "Okay. What's next on your list?" Most doctors appreciate that I've thought about the appointment ahead of time and structured our time together. It keeps both of us focused on the task at hand, and they know that when we're done with the list, we're done with the appointment.

Third, I learned in a book called *How Doctors Think* that most doctors decide on a diagnosis and treatment within minutes of seeing you. I think that my list makes them less likely to jump to a quick conclusion, because the list forces them to see me as more than a body "presenting" with a symptom.

Finally, my list makes me feel like an equal participant in the interaction; that alone increases the odds of a successful visit.

What if the doctor says, "I don't like lists"? Fine. Put it down. Here's your secret weapon though: be sure to memorize it before you go to the appointment. If the list is too long to memorize, it's too long for one appointment anyway.

Be sure to tell the doctor about any specialists you've seen or plan to see.

It's important to be on guard for what's called "care fragmentation." Unfortunately, this is becoming more and more common. You see a specialist about one particular symptom, and a different specialist about a different symptom, and maybe even a third specialist about a third symptom. However, the medical records that each doctor relies on don't contain information about the other appointments or their outcomes. I thought this problem would be solved when my records were put online; so far, that hasn't been the case.

I've been seeing a dermatologist about a skin condition for which she's prescribed a medication. During my appointments, after she examines me, she enters a lot of information on her computer. But whatever she's recording is not on the computer screen when my primary care doctor and I look at my medical records, even though the two doctors share the same health care facility. Where is the information she entered? I have no idea.

Care fragmentation can result in missed diagnoses: a skin rash being treated by a dermatologist could be related to joint pain being treated by a rheumatologist. My primary doctor wouldn't know about these other appointments unless I told him. I hope this changes soon.

Don't be afraid to ask questions.

I recommend going to every appointment with the assumption that the doctor is knowledgeable and is seeking the best outcome for you. That said, don't be shy about asking questions, including what alternative treatments might be available. If you take an ally with you, he or she can chime in should you forget to inquire about this. Doctors are often thinking about alternatives—just not out loud. When you ask questions, it encourages them to talk to you about what's going on in their heads—which is something you want to be a party to.

I don't recommend regaling the doctor with information from other sources (unless the doctor has encouraged you to do so). You're likely to lose a doctor's attention if you say, "Research on the internet shows… " If you have information that you think is important, share it in a way that communicates that you think of you and your doctor as partners in your health care. Hand it to the doctor, while saying something like "Doctor, I found this article that I thought might interest you" or "I know a lot of your patients must bring you material to read from the internet, but this particular article appears to be relevant to my condition. I'd love to get your feedback on it when you have time."

Repeat back your understanding of the plan of action.

When you sense your time is up, briefly describe your understanding of what has come out of the appointment. For example, you might say, "To be sure I understand you correctly, you want me to start this new medication, get a blood test in a week, and return in two weeks." I've had too many appointments where I get to the car afterward and neither my husband nor I can remember some important detail of what happened. The risk of this is even greater, of course, if you've gone to the appointment alone.

Don't write off a good doctor because of one disappointing visit.

Let me set the scene: You've seen this doctor before. The rapport was excellent. She was a good listener and involved you in the decision-making. You feel fortunate to be in her care. Then, out of the blue, you have an appointment at which she rushes you and isn't focusing on you as a flesh-and-blood person.

When this happened to me in the past, I'd jump to this conclusion: "My illness is too much of a hassle; she doesn't want me as her patient anymore." This reaction is an example of a type of distorted thinking called "overgeneralization." In this instance, I was taking one disappointing experience and drawing the general conclusion that all subsequent experiences with this doctor would be disappointing.

But life can be stressful for doctors too. This may have been a day when she was badly overbooked, or tired from lack of sleep, or worried about a family member. I used to feel personally hurt when a doctor with whom I had a good relationship wasn't as "present" for me as I'd become accustomed to. Over the years, I've learned that if I've already established a good relationship with a doctor, this reaction of mine is off the mark. Now I chalk my disappointment up to he or she having had an off day. In every instance so far, the next appointment has gone fine.

A disappointing visit might also be due to your doctor's frustration about not being able to "fix" you. Doctors learn in medical school: examine, diagnose, fix. However, that isn't how it goes for people who are chronically ill. If you have a good relationship with a doctor, I suggest that you give him or her some slack and accept that, some days, a hard-to-treat patient is too challenging for the doctor to handle gracefully.

I had an insight into this several years ago. I had a circular, itchy rash on my knee that wouldn't go away, so I made an appointment to see my primary care physician. He took a scraping and went off to look at it under a microscope. When he returned, he seemed so excited that I had something he could actually diagnose and fix that he took me down the hall to look through the microscope myself. He explained exactly what I was seeing: a simple fungus that was treatable with an over-the-counter ointment.

This interaction—seeing how happy he was to have *finally* been able to help me—gave me fresh insight into how difficult my illness must be for him at times. He's an exceptionally caring doctor, so it's understandable that once in a while he gets frustrated that he has a patient who's been sick since 2001 and that there's been little he's been able to do about it.

When things fall apart, cultivate equanimity.

Sometimes, despite your best effort, you may feel deflated—even inconsolable—when a doctor's appointment doesn't go well. I certainly have. This is a good time to cultivate equanimity: that mental calmness and evenness of temper that knows that sometimes things work out well and sometimes they don't. This is not a passive stance but an acknowledgment of the way things are. From this place of mental balance, and perhaps after a good cry, you can be proactive and take measured, concrete steps to improve the care you're getting (which may include finding another doctor) rather than lashing out in anger, which is unlikely to get you what you want or what you need.

21

Sick Upon Sick: Handling an Acute Illness While Chronically Ill

If you want real control, drop the illusion of control;
let life have you. It does anyway.

—BYRON KATIE

O CCASIONALLY, I come down with a viral or bacterial infection that's not related to my ongoing illness. It might be our familiar friend the common cold. It could be bronchitis or strep throat, or maybe that most unwelcome visitor—the bladder infection. I used to think of acute illnesses as minor irritations and nuisances. More often than not, they didn't even stop me from going to work. Now that I'm chronically ill, however, such illnesses are big events in my life. I call it "sick upon sick." In this chapter, I'll discuss the good, the bad, and the ugly of an acute illness settling in on top of a chronic one.

The Bad: Sleep Disruption

For most chronically ill people, a crucial indicator of how functional they'll be on any given day is how well they slept the night before. This is true for me. I can sleep well and still feel too sick to do much the next day, but if I *don't* sleep well, I'm guaranteed to feel too sick to do anything except rest in bed or on the couch. By contrast, when healthy people have a bad night's sleep, they feel crummy the next day, but they're still functional.

An acute illness almost always brings with it a bad night's sleep. Consider the effects of the common cold: a nose that alternates between being too stuffy to breathe through and too runny to contain; a tickly cough that seems to always kick in just as sleep is about to descend. Or strep throat: a throat so sore that the sensation of breath going across it can cause a wince. And why do bladder infections tend to show up in the middle of the night, assuring there will be no sleep from 2:00 a.m. on?

Sick upon sick: yuck! There's nothing to be done but follow Byron Katie's advice and let the new illness have me. It does anyway.

The Good: Forced Self-Care

Like almost every chronically ill person I know, I tend to push myself rather than stay strictly within limits that might help ease my symptoms. I'll do too much housework; I'll spend too much time visiting with a friend.

I can even push myself too far from the bed—at 4:00 a.m. while I'm still half asleep! Here's how. I'll become partially conscious and an idea for the book I'm working on will pop into my mind. Afraid that I'll forget it if I go back to sleep, I turn on the light and take a few notes. That, of course, wakes me up sufficiently that I can't get back to sleep.

When I have an acute illness, though, I take much better care of myself. A messy house is the last thing on my mind, and if I get one of those 4:00 a.m. ideas, I can't be bothered to try and get it down on paper. Instead, I say to myself: "If it's that important, I'll remember it later."

The Bad: Heightened Awareness of Isolation from Others

Isolation is such a challenge for the chronically ill that I devote a separate section in the book to it. I know how fortunate I am to have a live-in partner who loves me and takes good care of me. Aside from his company, my socializing is generally confined to short visits once a week with my friends Dawn and Richard, although sometimes I have to cancel with them.

When I have an acute illness, however, there's no question—I'm cancelling. For the most part, I no longer mind being alone so much of the time. Yet having a cold or another infection drives home how cut off I am from in-person contact. This heightened sense of isolation stems from realizing that, although the acute illness will go away, my limited ability to socialize with others will not. This adds emotional pain to the physical misery of whatever temporary symptoms I'm experiencing. As I'll discuss in the section on isolation, it's helpful to treat isolation as a companion. Maybe not a treasured companion, like Dawn and Richard, but a companion nonetheless on this chronic illness journey.

The Ugly: Worrying That What's Acute May Become Chronic

When the symptoms of an acute illness combine with the symptoms of a chronic illness, together they can feel like one big indistinguishable mess. When this happens to me, there's a nagging concern in the back of my mind that some of the new symptoms won't turn out to be acute; I worry that they'll hang around and become part of the constellation of my chronic symptoms.

To alleviate my worry, I keep a Don't-Know Mind. This is a

treasured practice from Korean Zen teacher Seung Sahn. He encouraged his students to keep a Don't-Know Mind about their views, about other people, and about the future. After all, do any of us know what will happen next in our lives?

Don't-Know Mind is one of my chronic illness survival tools. When I'm dealing with an acute illness, worrying about my symptoms can trigger a barrage of stressful stories. Keeping a Don't-Know Mind stops those stories in their tracks: "Will my throat hurt every time I inhale from now on?" *I don't know.* "Will I have a stuffy nose for the rest of my life?" *I don't know.* Don't-Know Mind has a calming effect, partly because it's so effective at revealing the absurdity of most of those stories. Do I really think my sore throat is permanent or that I'll have a stuffy nose for the rest of my life? No!

I can report this: so far, so good. When each acute episode has run its course, so have the symptoms that accompanied it.

The Good: Hope

Several doctors think that my continuing illness is due to my immune system being chronically activated. As one doctor put it, my immune system is "stuck in the 'on' position"—having never returned to normal after I got the acute viral infection in 2001. This means that, theoretically, something *could* come along that would "reset my immune system" (a phrase that several doctors have also used).

So whenever I get an acute illness, along with "The Bad" and "The Ugly," there's always the hope that when I recover, the acute illness will leave in its wake a normal immune system—and I'll no longer be sick! One of my doctors admitted to me that he hopes for the same thing whenever I'm "sick upon sick." It may never happen, so I don't get my expectations up. Nevertheless, a little hope creeps in every time.

Several years ago, I was getting acupuncture treatment—another hoped-for cure that didn't work out. One day I told the acupuncturist that I thought I was coming down with a cold. To my surprise, she brightened up and optimistically said to me, "There's a saying in Chinese medicine that you have to be well enough to get a cold." I never fail to remember her words when I get a cold—or any acute illness. The logic (or lack thereof) of this saying appeals to me, and it's a goofy enough idea that it just might be true.

It didn't come to pass with my last cold, but there's always the next one. Hope.

22

The Pesky Issue of Sleep

For you too, fleas,
the night must be long
it must be lonely.

—ISSA

CHRONIC ILLNESS can play havoc with those of us who try to follow traditional advice for good sleep. Hardly a week goes by without an article on proper sleep hygiene showing up during my internet wanderings. The recommendations may be good for some people; unfortunately they rarely work for a body that marches to the beat of chronic illness. In fact, some of them are downright irrelevant to our lives.

What follows is the conventional wisdom regarding sleep hygiene, along with my reflections on why it's unlikely to work for those of us who are chronically ill. This lighthearted analysis is based on my personal experience and on what others have told me. That said, if any of these traditional tips work for you, terrific. Keep following them!

Conventional wisdom: Don't use your bedroom for any activities other than sleeping or sex.

Yes, not just your bed, but your *bedroom*. The idea is to get your mind and body to associate the bedroom with sleep. Here are the types of activities on those "don't-do-in-the-bedroom" lists: talking on the phone, listening to the radio, watching television, reading, using the computer, and the big one—working.

The most prominent object in most bedrooms is the bed. Those of us who are chronically ill use it *a lot*. I wrote my first two books from the bed and I'm writing this one from the very same place. It's all happening in a four-foot-square space. I'd be able to call it a two-foot-square space except that my printer is four feet from the bed—still close enough, however, for me to reach with a good stretch of my left arm.

As you'll see in chapter 41, my bed is my office, my craft center, my entertainment center, my dog playground, my dining room. From my experience, I'd be hard-pressed to find a chronically ill person who only uses his or her bed for sleeping and for sex.

Conventional wisdom: Go to sleep at the same time every night.

I try. I really do try. Unfortunately, pain and other symptoms—not the clock—dictate when I'll be getting to sleep.

Conventional wisdom: Don't nap during the day.

According to the sleep hygiene experts, the reason for this rule is that napping will disrupt your natural patterns of sleep and wakefulness. Unfortunately, for the chronically ill, those natural patterns have already been disrupted.

As for me, I can't get through the day without a nap, not because I'm sleepy, but because after a certain amount of activity, my body breaks down the way a healthy person's body breaks down when he or she has the flu. I've tried going without a nap just to be sure it's necessary. The consequence is not a pretty sight. It's not pretty that afternoon, nor is it the next day when I'm still experiencing "payback" symptoms from my little adventure. Oh, and I consider it a small victory if I only need one nap. I've been known to need four.

Conventional wisdom: Aerobic exercise helps you sleep better.

Perhaps this would be true for me; I'll never know. As is the case for most people who are chronically ill, this kind of exercise is out of the question.

Conventional wisdom: Move the TV out of the bedroom.

This may be a good idea for some people, but if I didn't have a TV in the bedroom, I'd not have seen a single movie released since 2001, the year I got sick. The best I can do to accommodate this sleep hygiene rule is to turn the brightness way down on the television set. It doesn't make for great TV viewing for my husband; it's a good thing he's such an accommodating guy.

Conventional wisdom (and my personal favorite): If you don't fall asleep in 15-20 minutes, or if you wake up in the middle of the night and don't fall back asleep in 15-20 minutes, get out of bed, go into another room, do something nonstimulating for a half hour, and then try again.

First, I *never* fall asleep in 15–20 minutes. It takes me longer than that to get comfortable. Once I'm comfortable, I have to wait until the symptom parade calms down. On a good night, I'm asleep after about 45–60 minutes. On a bad night… well, let's not go there.

Second, (and this may be the most valuable piece of advice in this chapter), I've discovered that I feel much better the next day if I *don't* get out of bed when I wake up in the middle of the night and can't get back to sleep. Instead, I "fake sleep": I lie in bed in my usual sleep position and pretend to sleep. I've tried both—getting up versus fake sleeping. For me, the latter makes the day to come much more bearable. To my surprise, many people have written to me about the value of fake sleeping. And here I thought I'd invented it!

I've become so adept at fake sleeping that I've started fake napping. Some days, the severity of my symptoms keeps me from falling asleep during a nap. When this happens, I've discovered that it's better to lie still for an hour or two instead of getting up. My husband and I call this a "shutdown," as in "all systems are shut down, even though no sleep is taking place."

This chapter may be lighthearted in tone, but the issue of sleep is a serious one for the chronically ill. We wish the conventional wisdom regarding sleep hygiene worked for us; we'd be so much more functional if we could sleep better.

23

Longing for That Pre-Illness Life

The obstacle is the path.

—ZEN PROVERB

NOW AND THEN, I feel unsettled and edgy, but I can't put my finger on why. If I mindfully investigate how I'm feeling, it often turns out that the source of my uneasiness is a longing for my pre-illness life. None of us wants to get stuck in a painful longing for a life we can no longer lead, and none of us wants to get caught in the net of stressful emotions that tend to accompany that longing—emotions that include frustration, restlessness, and even anxiety. Yet sometimes that's exactly what happens: we find ourselves stuck in a longing that simply cannot be satisfied.

The Vietnamese Zen monk and teacher Thich Nhat Hanh said: "Awareness is like the sun. When it shines on things, they are transformed." When I expose this longing for my pre-illness life to the sunlight of mindful awareness, I can begin to work skillfully with it. I start by giving myself a dose of reality: "You're in a body, and bodies get sick and injured. It happens to everyone. This is how it's happened to you. No amount of wishing it were otherwise is going to change that."

Then I take a deep breath—a sigh, really—and let the longing be. Yes, I *let it be*. I don't try to force it away, because that tends to set up a stubborn resistance in my mind. I simply let it be, with compassion for how hard it is to be missing my old life. As I let it be, I reflect on impermanence. Thoughts and emotions arise; thoughts and emotions pass away. If I'm patient, I know that the longing will subside, even though it may return to visit on another day.

As you read through this chapter, I hope you'll keep in mind our tendency to put the past on a pedestal. My life before I got sick wasn't always pleasant. It had its good times and its tough times. That said, here's a sampling of what I miss most about my life before chronic illness. Some of these I've managed to find substitutes for; others have been lost. Based on the many emails and other communications I get from people who are chronically ill, this list will be familiar.

The ability to be spontaneous.

Having to plan everything out in detail is rarely fun. Having to then impose those detailed plans on others is *never* fun. In the fall of 2013, my brother-in-law and his wife drove from about an hour away to have dinner with us. It would have been nice if we could have said to them: "Come any time in the afternoon; we'll hang out and then eat a leisurely dinner." Unfortunately, we couldn't offer such an open-ended invitation; it simply won't work for me.

If I visit in the afternoon, I won't be able to join them for dinner. And if they only come for dinner, it had better be an early one because at about 7:00, I turn into a pumpkin, as we put it in our household. So they came at 4:30, and we ate dinner at 5:30. It was great to see them, even though there was nothing spontaneous about the occasion—at least not to me.

If people unexpectedly call and say they're in town and would like to come over, whether I can visit depends entirely on the timing. I can't get through the day without a nap—and then, of course, there's that turning into a pumpkin by early evening. Truth be told, unless my husband is home, I rarely say it's okay for people to come over. This is because, if he's home, I know I can disappear into the bedroom if I have to. Not that this feels good to me—it can feel as if I'm hiding out from the very people I want to see. Many a tear has been shed in my bedroom over my inability to be spontaneous when it comes to socializing.

Then there's the lack of spontaneity when something comes up on the spur-of-the-moment. One day, my husband said, "Hey, *Lincoln* is playing in town. I'd love to see it!" And I thought, "I'd love to go with him." Then that dose-of-reality voice took over: "Hmm. It's two-and-a-half hours long, so with the previews and ads, that's closing in on three hours—much longer than I can sit up for. When I face that kind of wait at a doctor's office, I have to ask for a room to lie down in. I'll not be going to *Lincoln*."

This inability to be spontaneous impacts our loved ones too. When I decline someone's offer to come over for a visit, it cuts my husband off socially as well. And as for movies: if he wants to go to one, unless he's out-of-town, visiting family, he goes alone.

Variety.

They say variety is the spice of life. If so, my spice rack is pretty bare. I'm not complaining. It's just the way things are. I know how fortunate I am to live in a comfortable house with a loving partner, but still, every day is much the same for me. Some days, that "sameness" can get me down. My husband and I don't even have the questionable luxury of dealing with variety in my health issues.

Because my condition has remained almost unchanged since 2001, conversations between us about my health cover the same territory, over and over again.

I miss the variety that comes from seeing different people. As a teacher, I used to stare out over a sea of as many as a hundred different faces at one time. And when I wasn't in the classroom, I was a people watcher. Sometimes at restaurants I'd imagine a "back story" to the lives of those I'd be watching. Now I pretty much see the same people every day—and I already know their back stories.

When I feel sad about my inability to be spontaneous or about the lack of variety in my life, I begin by evoking compassion for myself; I gently remind myself that life can be hard at times, and that losses like these can be painful. Then I cultivate equanimity by reminding myself that everyone's life is a mixture of joys and sorrows, and that I feel better when I make peace with my disappointments, first by gently acknowledging them and then by allowing acceptance to settle in at its own pace.

Being actively involved in the life of my family.

I miss socializing in general, but what I miss most is being active in the life of my family. I miss the joy of having all of us gather together at the same time. I miss going to my two granddaughters' special events, such as Malia's dance shows and Cam's Little League games. But mostly, I wish I could take the two of them on little outings. One day in 2012, my husband took the hour drive to our granddaughter Cam's house for the sole purpose of driving her across the Bay Bridge so they could ride a cable car together in San Francisco.

That's what I miss.

Time in nature.

Some people who are chronically ill may miss hiking in the wilderness. My time in nature was more tame; I spent a lot of it in the arboretum at the University of California–Davis. The arboretum sits next to the law school building where I worked, and I walked the paths that line its creek almost every day. I knew every plant and tree and how they looked during each of the four seasons. I knew where the little green heron would be watching for fish and where the turtles would be sunning themselves on the banks of the creek.

My backyard has become my substitute for those forays into nature. I've become acutely aware of the four seasons moving through the deciduous trees that I see through my bedroom window—a mulberry, an elm, and a fig tree. Until I became sick, I didn't know what a prize those figs were for the birds in my neighborhood.

The ability to pursue my former interests.

Perhaps you were an active outdoors person or an avid moviegoer or a social activist. Maybe you loved to exercise or dance. One of my favorite pastimes was birdwatching. I particularly loved to spot shorebirds at marshlands and at the beach. I had a journal in which I recorded each sighting: the place, the day and time, the type of bird. From a friend who was an expert birder, I learned that the best way to identify a bird was to memorize a unique marking that I could then look up later in one of my bird books. If I still didn't know what it was, it went down in my journal as an LBJ, a designation taught to me by another birder-friend: Little Brown Job. (Were I able to go birding today, I'd probably identify birds on the spot by using an app on my smartphone!)

I don't see shorebirds anymore, but I'm learning to appreciate the beauty I'd taken for granted that's within eyeshot of my house: white-crowned sparrows, house finches, and the occasional hermit thrush in winter; doves and robins in spring; a quick fly-through of cedar waxwings if I can catch them; scrub jays and mockingbirds year-round.

Scrub jays are so common in California's Central Valley (we call them scrubbers) that I forget how stunning they are. Sometimes I treat a scrubber as a rare sighting by pretending I've never seen one before. Every time I do this, I'm amazed anew by the beauty of its iridescent bright blue and silver coloring.

Helping people out face-to-face.

Before I got sick, I was a court-appointed mentor for a boy in Child Protective Services. I was allowed to see him once a week. I'd pick him up at the home for emotionally disturbed boys where he lived, and we'd go out to dinner and then do something fun together. The two of us grew very close. I still feel bad that I couldn't continue to be a part of his life after I got sick (we weren't allowed to give our address or phone number to our child). And although it's been many years, I occasionally worry that he felt abandoned by me, even though his caseworker and I did our best to explain to him what happened to me.

I miss this kind of in-person interaction. It made me feel as if I were making life better for someone I cared deeply about. As is true for many people who are housebound by chronic pain and illness, I've turned to the internet. I'm grateful it has allowed me to continue to try and make a positive difference in people's lives.

Puttering around the house, doing my favorite things.

I loved to garden and occasionally still do some light pruning. Other than that, the little gardening I'm able to do is confined to pulling weeds—because they're what inevitably catch my eye when I go outside.

I also loved to paint rooms. Perhaps this was a holdover from my days as an undergraduate in college when I painted houses as a summer job. This was one of my joys as a homeowner: paint a room one color and then… paint it another! Now I'm in a bedroom that badly needs painting—as well as a new rug—but I haven't the ability to do what needs to be done; the preparation and then the disruption would be more than I can handle. The rug can be replaced… but can I handle being displaced? We're considering it.

My health not being the elephant in the room.

We've all had the experience of being with others when there's an issue looming large; everyone is aware of it but nobody wants to talk about it. I miss visiting with people without the state of my health being that issue.

This can get complicated and stressful for me. For starters, I never know if others will express an interest in how I'm doing or in what treatments I'm trying. Nor do I know whether they'll even acknowledge my condition with a simple "I'm sorry you're sick." But if they *don't* mention my health, I can't know if it's because they're uncomfortable raising it or if it's because they're assuming I'll bring it up if I want to talk about it.

Any way I look at it, I miss being around others without constantly wondering whether the issue of my health will become a topic of conversation and, if it does, how best to handle it.

The Zen proverb that starts this chapter says, "The obstacle is the path." For the chronically ill, longing for the life we can no longer lead can feel like an insurmountable obstacle. Sometimes the things I loved to do before I got sick feel as if they're dangling in front of me like carrots on a stick.

Looked at another way, however, this is my path. As I noted at the beginning of this chapter, when I'm caught in a painful longing to have my pre-illness life back, I don't try to force it away. But I do see it as an opportunity to practice being at peace with what I have right here, right now, even if it's not what I ordered up. I don't always succeed in this practice, but when I do, I know I'm resting in the peace of equanimity.

24
The Uncertainty of It All

Simply be present with your own shifting energies and
with the unpredictability of life as it unfolds.
—PEMA CHÖDRÖN

I'VE MADE repeated references in this book to one of the realities of the human condition: impermanence. It's a universal law, recognized in spiritual and scientific traditions alike. Everything is in flux from moment-to-moment, including our physical and mental states.

I like to think of uncertainty as a corollary of the universal law of impermanence. If everything is impermanent, then our lives and the people in it are uncertain—as well as unpredictable.

It's natural for us to wish things were otherwise. If we knew with certainty how each day was going to unfold, we'd feel safer and more secure. But all our wishing won't make it so. Uncertainty is a fact of life, whether we live in a third-world country or in the most advanced scientific and technological environment, and whether we're struggling to make ends meet or living in the lap of luxury.

For the chronically ill, life's unpredictability can feel as if it's increased exponentially. Indeed, perhaps the hardest thing about being chronically ill is the extra dose of uncertainty it brings to almost every aspect of our lives.

Uncertainty about how we'll feel on any given day... or even at any given moment.

For the chronically ill, not knowing how sick we'll feel or how much pain we'll be in makes it difficult to make plans. Because my symptoms can change at any moment, even after I've woken up, I don't know how I'll feel as the day progresses. Trying to plan ahead by resting for days in advance of an event doesn't necessarily help; I still may not feel good enough to participate when the day arrives.

At times, the unpredictability of my symptoms has been such a source of unhappiness that I've directed angry frustration at myself, as though it were my fault that I couldn't control the moment-to-moment course of this illness. I've been working on shedding this self-blame by reminding myself that whatever symptoms happen to be present at the moment are due to the vagaries of the illness.

In other words, I'm learning not to take symptoms personally. Inspired by a teaching from the Buddha, I consciously practice this by treating how I'm feeling at any given moment as being the result of the temporary coming together of causes and conditions in my life that are almost always out of my control. To do this, I intentionally omit self-referential terms, such as "I," "me," and "mine" from my thinking. After all, when causes and conditions come together to create aches and pains in my body, it's not as if I, Toni Bernhard, intentionally ordered up these unpleasant physical sensations!

It's the same with any symptoms that accompany chronic illness. Thinking of them as "me" or "mine" makes us feel as if we're responsible for their presence. The skillful and compassionate alternative is to regard fluctuating symptoms as part of the uncertainty and unpredictability that is inherent in all of life.

Here's an example of how this practice works. When pain is present, instead of thinking "I'm in miserable pain," I purposefully omit "I'm" and change the thought to "Pain is present" or "Pain is happening." I also use this practice with the stressful emotions that often accompany physical discomfort. And so, instead of thinking "I'm anxious about how long this pain will last," I purposefully omit "I'm" and change the thought to "Anxiety is present" or "Anxiety is happening." Same with frustration: "Frustration is present" or "Frustration is happening."

When I change the description of my experience in this way, it's easier to accept the uncertainty and unpredictability of how I'll feel on any particular day or at any given moment. This helps me to not take personally either physical discomfort or the stressful emotions that can accompany it. Instead, I regard them both as having arisen as the result of causes and conditions that happen to be present at this point in time.

I hope you'll try this. Taking self-referential terms out of the description of how you're feeling, physically and emotionally, can help you cope better "with the unpredictability of life as it unfolds," as Pema Chödrön put it. Pain is just happening. Deepseated fatigue is just happening. Heart palpitations are just happening. Frustration is just happening. Anxiety is just happening. None of this need be taken personally. It's just how life is for you at the moment.

With your mind feeling more at ease from this practice, you can shift your focus to the peaceful abiding of equanimity, which means accepting as best you can that life will always be uncertain: these are the physical symptoms and the mind states that are present right now, and you can't predict what the next moment might bring. No one can.

Uncertainty about what social commitments to make.

Not overcommitting ourselves while also not unnecessarily isolating ourselves from others is a delicate balancing act. These mental gymnastics can be exhausting for us. For me, they begin as soon as someone asks if he or she can come over for a visit. If I say yes, how do I know I'll be well enough to keep the commitment when the day arrives? This tips the scales in favor of saying no, so that I don't have to cancel on short notice. On the other hand, if I say no and then feel well enough to visit on that day, I've passed up the opportunity to be in the good company of another person. Managing chronic illness is hard—and often exhausting—work.

In the end, when the opportunity to socialize arises, each of us has to decide what to do, based on our mindful assessment of how we're feeling. We should then resolve not to blame ourselves if it turns out we made the wrong choice; that's self-compassion in action. In my case, because I never have a day when I don't feel sick, I tend to choose the safe alternative and decline the offer of a visit, even though this may mean that I'm more isolated than I need be.

And what about a social commitment that would have too many negative ramifications were we to cancel? If I'm feeling particularly sick on a day when this is the case, I find it helpful to say to myself, "Whether you feel your *usual* sick self or your *extra* sick self, this is something you have to do, so do it as graciously and with as little complaining as possible."

Uncertainty about how others will treat us.

We're never sure how family and friends—and, of course, doctors—will react to our illness and to our pain. I've experienced both extremes: people pulling away from me in aversion and others embracing me with compassion. It also feels as if I've experienced everything in between. I've had people talk to me as if I'm a child. I've had people speak to me in a pitying voice. I've had people drill me with questions about my illness as if I'm on the witness stand. I've had others speak to me with genuine concern. I've had people utter those most welcomed words: "I'm sorry you're sick."

Uncertainty about how people might treat me used to give rise to such severe stress that, before seeing someone, my heart would begin to race and my face would get flushed. I've learned, however, that even well-intentioned people often behave unskillfully. Our culture does a poor job of teaching people about chronic illness. Recognizing that unskilled speech is usually the result of ignorance on the part of the speaker helps me not to take his or her behavior personally.

I've found that the best way to handle uncertainty about how people will react to my chronic condition is to put aside my expectations and keep what I referred to in chapter 21 as a "Don't-Know Mind." I don't expect people *to* understand… and I don't expect people *not* to understand. I just hope for the best, and I try to respond to them as honestly and as graciously as I can under the circumstances.

Uncertainty about how much help we should ask for.

A few years ago, my husband was making plans to leave town for two weeks. He asked me what he should stock up on from the grocery store. I told him not to bother because I was feeling well enough to go to the store myself. Unfortunately, I'd forgotten how much energy it takes to do the household tasks that he handles when he's at home. As a result, I wasn't well enough to go to the store. For five days, the only veggie I ate was spinach. Then my neighbor Nadine learned from one of my Facebook posts that I was home alone. She asked if I'd like her to go to the store for me. Needless to say, I jumped at her kind offer.

Because our ability to do things for ourselves on any given day is uncertain and unpredictable, it's hard to know how much help to line up ahead of time. We don't want to burden family and friends with tasks if we can do them ourselves, especially because most of us value our independence. On the other hand, neither do we want our cupboards to be bare because we overestimated how much we could do for ourselves.

Uncertainty about how we'll react to a routine medical procedure.

Whether healthy or not, no one looks forward to getting a root canal. Then there's that lovely procedure known as the colonoscopy. At least people in good health have a decent idea of what side effects to expect. For the chronically ill, however, a routine procedure can trigger a flare in symptoms that may take days or weeks to recover from.

This unpredictability about how we'll react to medical procedures can have serious consequences. I know I'm not alone among the chronically ill in putting off routine procedures because I'm uncertain about how I'll react to them. The only one I'm diligent about is the colonoscopy because my mother had colon cancer. Fear trumps uncertainty in that instance.

I've learned that the best way to handle a colonoscopy, or any procedure I'm concerned about, is to acknowledge with compassion for myself the stress I'm feeling. I also remind myself that this is important self-care—important for maintaining what I think of as "wellness within illness."

(Note to self: must stop cancelling and rescheduling—over and over again—those routine dental cleanings.)

Uncertainty about our ability to handle an emergency.

Uncertainty about how I'll be able to cope in an emergency is one of the most stressful challenges I've faced since becoming ill in 2001. At times it's given rise to intense worry and fear. I particularly agonize over what would happen should my own caregiver need a caregiver.

In April of 2013, I had a taste of what would happen in an emergency. I learned from the experience that, although I have the ability to step up in the short term if I need to, there's a limit to how long I can sustain that type of behavior.

One morning, my husband had a severe allergic reaction (probably to something he ate). When the reaction set in, I drove him to the emergency room, which is about ten minutes from our house. Once we got there, I sat by his bed as they hooked him up to an IV and put an oxygen mask on him. Then I waited as he lay there, barely conscious and unable to communicate with me.

In addition to being worried about him, I was concerned about the limitations imposed by my illness. With great effort, I can manage to sit in a chair for about two hours before I feel as if I'm going to keel over. As I sat there, I had no idea what time frame we were looking at. Would we be there for an hour or for six hours? (It turned out to be the latter.)

After two hours, I could barely sit upright in the chair. I told the nurse that I suffered from a chronic illness and needed to lie down for a short time. She politely told me that I should go home and call them in a couple of hours to see how my husband was doing. No way! I wasn't going to leave him alone when he'd yet to respond to treatment. Not knowing what else to do, I called our friend Richard. When he arrived, I left him in the room with my husband and went out to our van to lie down for a while.

As I lay there, I felt as if my life had come to a sorry state. Here

I was, in a parking lot, lying on our dog's hair-covered and not-so-fragrant blanket, pulling whatever I could find over me in order to keep warm (including newspapers), using my lumpy purse as a pillow. When I returned to the ER, my husband had his eyes open and was no longer disoriented. After another two hours, they discharged him, and I drove us home.

Once I felt confident that he'd be okay, I became acutely aware that this emergency room adventure had brought my limitations into sharp focus. What if I needed to be at his bedside in the hospital for days at a time? What if he developed a chronic medical problem and needed a caregiver of his own to take over the household tasks? Should I even be spending time fretting about events that may never materialize?

Since that day in 2013, I've thought a lot about what I can and cannot handle in an emergency. I'm trying to walk a middle path. On the one hand, I don't want to ruin my present-moment experience by spending all my time worrying about my ability to handle an emergency; after all, an event like this may never happen again. On the other hand, I realize that it's important for me and my husband to plan for some very real possibilities that could be beyond my ability to manage.

Living at ease with life's uncertainty is difficult enough without the added challenge of chronic illness. Will we ever be able to do the things we treasured so much before we got sick? Will the people we meet treat us with understanding and compassion? What does the future hold? We just don't know.

Since uncertainty is an inevitable part of the human experience, the quality of our lives will improve dramatically if we can find a way to make peace with it. When I awake each morning, I try to remember to reflect on how I can't know what the day has in store for me, especially with regard to my health. Then I set the intention to greet it nonetheless with as much caring attention, compassion, and open-hearted curiosity as I can muster. I hope you'll do the same.

25

Taking Care of the Caregivers

*The most precious gift we can offer anyone is
our presence. When our mindfulness embraces those
we love, they will bloom like flowers.*

—THICH NHAT HANH

M Y CAREGIVER has had a front-row seat for chronic illness
since 2001. But I've had a front-row seat too: watching the
life of the caregiver. I've learned that the difficulties he faces are as
great as mine, although he might not agree with me.

In the study "Quality of Life: Impact of Chronic Illness on the
Partner," published in the *Journal of the Royal Society of Medicine*
in November 2001, the authors reported:

> The most striking research finding is a tendency for the
> partner's quality of life to be worse than that of the
> patient.

Although the study focused on partners and spouses, I expect that its findings would be similar when the relationship of caregiver and cared-for person is parent/child, child/parent, sibling/sibling, or a host of other relationships. I know three parents who are caregivers for chronically ill young children. There's no doubt that these parents' quality of life has suffered, partly due to their extra responsibilities (which includes making sure their children get a proper education) and partly because of their ongoing worries about how their children will fare physically, emotionally, and socially. The need to care for a child can also impact their ability to climb the career ladder or even force them to give up their careers altogether.

This chapter offers suggestions for taking care of caregivers. It focuses on caregivers who are spouses or partners, but it applies to anyone who is taking care of a loved one. I'll begin with how the person who is being cared for can help. Then I'll cover how family members and friends can help. A theme that runs throughout the chapter is that the best way to take care of caregivers is to give them your loving and caring attention.

If You're the One Being Cared For

Talk with your caregiver about what's reasonable for him or her to do for you, what you can do for yourself, and what you both need help with.

Most caregivers have commitments that aren't related to their caregiving duties. Their most crucial commitment may be holding down a job in order to support the family. That alone can take up most of their day. Taking into consideration these noncaregiving responsibilities, have a heart-to-heart talk with your caregiver about what he or she can reasonably do for you.

If you don't have this conversation, your caregiver is likely to think that he or she has to do everything. This can quickly lead to caregiver burnout and even to clinical depression; both of these are common consequences of being overwhelmed as a caregiver. Taking on too much responsibility can also compromise your caregiver's physical health.

Once you've agreed on what's reasonable for your caregiver to do for you, talk about what you can usually do for yourself and also about who you'd be comfortable turning to for help with other tasks. In our household, my husband takes care of the finances, and he does the shopping, the cooking, the dishes, and his own laundry. In addition, he runs all the errands and takes care of car maintenance. Oh, and he's my computer help desk.

On my end, I wash my own clothes, feed the dog, and try to keep the house from getting too cluttered. I also arrange for people to come over when something in the house needs repairing or replacing and when the yard needs special maintenance, such as tree trimming. Then, when they come to the house, if at all possible, I handle the interactions. Sometimes this takes me beyond my limits (especially if they're chatty!) and, as a result, my symptoms flare. I do it anyway because I want to protect my husband from caregiver burnout.

Once you and your caregiver have decided what the two of you can reasonably handle, you'll be in a position to assess what kind of help you'll need from others. I sometimes need a ride to a doctor's or lab appointment. My husband sometimes needs a friend to come with him on a two-person errand, as he did when he picked up our new puppy, who was on a ranch that's a two-and-a-half-hour drive from where we live.

To brush up on your "asking for help" skills, I suggest you review chapter 3, "Asking for Help Can Be Your Gift to Others." Many of us have been taught that it's a sign of weakness to ask for help. It's not. When someone asks for my help, I've never thought, "Oh, she's weak!" In addition, we tend to assume that if people wanted to help, they'd have come forward and offered. It took several years for me to realize that people wanted to lend a hand but needed to be asked. Once asked, they jumped at the opportunity.

Find ways to preserve your pre-illness relationship.

Think about what you and your caregiver have enjoyed in the past about being in each other's company. This is a mindfulness practice. Take some time to consciously pay attention to what made your relationship "tick." Then make a commitment to nourish that part of the relationship. Doing this can improve both your and your caregiver's quality of life.

Perhaps you loved laughing together. If so, think about how you can do that in a way that doesn't push you beyond your limitations. Maybe you can't go to a comedy club, but you could watch your favorite stand-up comedians in concert on a television or computer screen.

Sometimes my husband and I play Scrabble with each other on our computers. He sits on the bed next to me while I'm lying down. We each have the Scrabble game open on our laptops. When he plays his letters, there's a slight pause and then an audible "ping" as his move pops up on my computer. It may seem as if this lacks the personal connection of sitting opposite each other over a Scrabble board, but it doesn't. For us, online Scrabble is as enjoyable as the traditional way of playing, and it's the only way we *can* play because I can't sit upright at a table long enough to complete a game.

Perhaps you and your caregiver liked to talk about certain subjects: politics, for instance, or your spiritual life. Pick the time of day when you have the most energy and try to engage your caregiver in a lively conversation.

Preserving the relationship you had with your caregiver before you became chronically ill may require careful planning. It's worth the effort, though, because it provides the opportunity to do something emotionally nourishing and enjoyable for both of you. Perhaps the best reward for your effort will be that you'll finally be doing something together that has nothing to do with the state of your health!

Encourage your caregiver to do things without you.

Caregivers can be reluctant to do enjoyable things for themselves. They may feel that if they don't treat taking care of you as a full-time commitment, they're falling short as a caregiver. They may also feel that they shouldn't be doing something that's fun if you can't join in. But I want my husband to enjoy himself. It's good for his mental and physical health, and it makes it easier for me to feel okay about how much of his time is devoted to my care.

I hope you'll encourage your caregiver to go to dinner with a friend, take in a movie, pursue a hobby, or even just read a good book. If your caregiver brushes aside your suggestions, let him or her know that it would be good for both of you. Say something like "This is what I want for you. Not only that, but I feel better when I know you're enjoying yourself."

If your caregiver is housebound much of the time because of the need to be close by, help him or her find new ways to do old things. For example, a caregiver can stay connected to other people through Skype or FaceTime. My husband and our granddaughter Malia love sending each other photos or short videos through Snapchat.

It's good for both of you if your caregiver's life is not solely about caring for you. With compassion in your heart for all he or she does for you, take the lead in encouraging your caregiver to have some fun.

Be sure you're not taking your caregiver for granted.

Mindfulness is helpful here. Are you paying careful attention to everything your caregiver does for you? I've noticed that I can get complacent. I'll passively accept a meal that my husband has cooked, or I'll mumble "thanks" when he brings me a prescription he's picked up from the pharmacy—a trip he wouldn't have had to make were I healthy.

When I realize that I'm beginning to take him for granted, I immediately tell him how much I appreciate him. If he shrugs it off like it's no big deal, I respond by ticking off his duties, one by one, to remind him of the tasks he's had to take on. I want to be sure he remembers that not all spouses or loved ones have the extra responsibilities he does. I certainly don't have them!

Every little thing your caregiver does for you is a gift. You can return that gift by making sure your caregiver knows how much you value what he or she does for you—day in and day out.

Remind your caregiver that your health might improve.

I've improved a bit since the early years of my illness. Although I still can't travel, I am able to spend more time out of the bedroom. Sometimes I'm able to go a café in the afternoon or out to an early dinner. By contrast, those first few years, I was completely bedbound and unable to socialize with family or friends when they came over.

I often have to remind myself how much worse those first years were; it's so easy to see the glass as half empty as opposed to half full. These small changes in my health have made my husband's life easier and more enjoyable. For this reason, it's good to remind your caregiver that it's possible your condition might improve. As

I like to put it: sometimes the universal law of impermanence can be our friend.

Help your caregiver accept your new life and even see the positives in it.

Whether or not your health changes for the better, you and your caregiver can work on making peace with your life as it is at the moment. You could gently remind your caregiver that people's lives sometimes take unexpected and unwelcome turns. Life is uncertain and unpredictable for everyone. Even though this is not how both of you hoped to be spending these years, it's what the two of you have. The more you can accept it without bitterness, the more peace of mind you'll find.

My husband and I have an exchange that I think of as our little equanimity practice. Once in a while, I say to him, sincerely but matter-of-factly, "I wish I weren't sick"; he then says to me in the same neutral, nonaversive tone, "I wish you weren't sick." Then we get on with our lives—however that life is at the moment.

You can also make a conscious effort to consider the unexpected blessings this new life has brought to both of you, such as the opportunity to spend more time together or the chance to take up a new hobby. Maybe it's been your ticket out of the rat race! Whatever benefits you can think of, share them with your caregiver and, together, treasure and nourish them.

Don't let red flags about your caregiver's own health go unheeded.

It's not unusual for caregivers to ignore any symptoms they develop so long as those symptoms aren't as severe as yours. Please don't hesitate to push your caregiver to seek medical attention when you think he or she needs it. And when your caregiver *is* being treated for something, even if it's minor, don't forget to ask how he or she is doing. Since becoming my caregiver, my husband has never had so much attention from me over a stubbed toe!

If You're the Friend or Family Member of a Caregiver

Be ready to talk about things that aren't related to his or her caregiver duties.

Of course, if a caregiver wants to talk about the difficulties he or she is facing with caregiving, be a good and compassionate listener. Most caregivers, however, will also welcome the opportunity to talk about something other than their loved one's health. I know my husband appreciates it when people raise other subjects.

I've learned from him that my ongoing illness can be a conversation killer. When he's with other people and the state of my health comes up, after he reports "She's about the same," no one feels it would be appropriate to say "How about those Giants!" The ideal way for people to respond would be to say something like "Please give Toni my best" and then change the subject to something of mutual interest. Most caregivers would be relieved to engage with someone on a topic—almost any topic—that's not health-related!

Invite a caregiver to do something with you, even if it's an activity you used to do with the caregiver and the person in his or her care.

My husband and I have noticed that people will invite a single friend over for dinner or to join them in an activity, and yet they rarely invite a spouse or a partner who is a caregiver. This has the effect of increasing a caregiver's social isolation. People have good intentions. Often, they simply assume that he wouldn't want to come without me. Other times, they're concerned that I'll feel bad that I've been left out.

If you're a friend or family member of a caregiver, please include him or her, particularly on special occasions. Let the caregiver know that you're aware that he or she may have to come alone, and that it's fine with you. Recently, a friend of ours invited my husband to her baby shower. How thoughtful!

Offer specific help.

This suggestion also appears in the chapter on what the chronically ill hope others will say to them. As is true for a person who is chronically ill, a caregiver is unlikely to follow-up on an open-ended offer such as "Call me if there's anything I can do for you" or "I wish there were something I could do to help." On the other hand, if you're going to the hardware store, a caregiver would welcome a call in which you ask if there's anything you can pick up.

Even better, offer to give the caregiver a break by taking care of his or her children for a few hours or by offering to do one of those seemingly minor tasks that add up fast, such as mowing the lawn or washing the car.

Studying my husband as caregiver, I've learned that many of the difficulties we face overlap: we've both become isolated socially; we've both lost each other's company as travel companions (as I'm writing this, he's alone in the car on the six-hour drive to visit our daughter's family for the weekend); we both face a lack of understanding from others about the effects of chronic illness on everyday life; we've both spent inordinate amounts of time in health care facilities; we both face uncertainty about what will happen if he should need someone to care for him.

In addition to the challenges they share with the person in their care, caregivers face their own set of stressors. They must live with the frustration and helplessness of not being able to make their loved one better. They've been thrust into the role of patient advocate in the medical system, a role for which they have neither training nor expertise. They often have to take over the running of the household.

Finally, they're the ones who see their loved one at his or her very worst. When I'm in the company of others, I do my best to appear energetic and socially engaged. This takes adrenaline, and the devastating after-effects this can have on me are for my husband's eyes and ears only. When we're alone again, it's he who must deal with the physical and emotional fallout from my having overextended myself around others. I'm positive that this is a familiar scenario to most of you who are reading this.

Caregivers are in need of care too. They know when a person is paying attention to their concerns and their needs, and they appreciate it greatly. Reaching out with compassion to ease their burden can improve the quality of life for these unsung heroes in the world of the chronically ill.

Feeling heard and understood is as important to a caregiver as it is to the person in his or her care.

V. Isolation and Loneliness

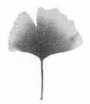

26

Quotations and Reflections on Loneliness

Only the lonely know the way I feel tonight.
—ROY ORBISON

CHRONIC ILLNESS can bring with it a dramatic change in life-style. It did for me. Before I got sick, I spent my days in the company of others. Sometimes I had over a hundred students in my classroom. My husband and I were active in our community, attending social and cultural events almost every weekend. Then I got sick, and suddenly I was alone much of the time. I'm still working on how to be alone without being lonely.

I take comfort in Roy Orbison's lyrics. They're a reminder that when loneliness descends on me, at least I know there are others who understand how I feel; that, in itself, makes me feel less lonely. I'm hoping these quotations and reflections will help you feel more connected to others and will point the way toward learning to be alone without feeling lonely.

Language... has created the word "loneliness" to express
the pain of being alone. And it has created the word "solitude"
to express the glory of being alone.

—PAUL TILLICH

When I first saw this quotation, I was confused because I'd always equated being alone with loneliness. I've since learned that Tillich is right. Being alone, in itself, is a neutral state—neither negative nor positive. It becomes emotionally painful when we add to it an intense longing for circumstances over which we have no control to be different than they are. When that longing goes unsatisfied, being alone turns into Tillich's painful loneliness.

If we open our hearts and minds to look for what we might treasure about being alone, it can become Tillich's glorious solitude. The chapters in this section explore how we might do this.

The real loneliness is living among all these kind people
who only ask one to pretend.

—EDITH WHARTON, *The Age of Innocence*

Everyone has had the experience of being in the presence of "kind people who only ask one to pretend"; the chronically ill are often expected to pretend to be healthy. I used to be hurt when I perceived that the people I'm closest to were asking this of me, and sometimes I'd feel disappointed and even angry at them once I was out of their company. Now I try to see it from their point of view. I believe that their heartfelt wish for me to be healthy can be so overwhelming at times that it leads them to pretend that I *am* healthy... and to expect me to pretend with them.

Music was my refuge. I could crawl into the spaces between
the notes and curl my back to loneliness.
—MAYA ANGELOU

I love Angelou's image of curling her back to loneliness—nestling into the spaces between the notes until the fit was so snug that music was the only thing that could get through to fill her heart.

Your refuge need not be music. It can be anything that brings you comfort—a cuddly pet or even a special pillow. The audiobooks of E. M. Forster and Alexander McCall Smith serve that purpose for me. The narrators are like old friends; I feel cozy and protected in their presence. I curl my back to loneliness by listening to the same books over and over, just as Angelou must have done with her favorite pieces of music.

Remember we're all in this alone.
—LILY TOMLIN

I can always count on Lily to bring a smile to my face and take me out of my self-focused thinking.

I felt a haunting loneliness sometimes, and felt it in others...
young clerks in the dusk, wasting the most poignant moments
of night and life.
—F. SCOTT FITZGERALD, *The Great Gatsby*

Fitzgerald is reminding us that loneliness is not always confined to the bed or the house—or even to being alone. Some people who work all day around others feel terribly lonely. We shouldn't assume that loneliness is the prerogative of those who are isolated by chronic illness or other circumstances.

*Inside myself is a place where I live all alone and that's where
you renew your springs that never dry up.*
—PEARL S. BUCK

Had I not become chronically ill, I might never have understood what Pearl S. Buck was saying; before I got sick, I was around other people most of the time and rarely paid attention to what was going on inside me. Now that I'm alone a lot, if I turn my attention inward and listen carefully, I can hear the trickling of that spring—fresh and full of promise. It is, indeed, a moment of renewal, one in which I'm content to watch—in the words of the poet Mary Oliver—my "one wild and precious life" unfold.

*Loneliness adds beauty to life. It puts a special burn
on sunsets and makes night air smell better.*
—HENRY ROLLINS

I can't yet claim that loneliness adds beauty to my life, but I have experienced a bittersweet quality to it. Perhaps this is what Rollins is referring to. When my husband is away for several days or weeks, loneliness can settle in. It's bitter in that I'd love to share with another person the sight of the clouds setting up for a beautiful sunset, as is so often the case outside my living room window. It's bitter in that it would feel good to take in the aroma of the night air with someone by my side. Yet, when I'm alone, there's also a sweetness in the heightened sense of awareness of what's going on around me, a sweetness that brings with it appreciation of that "special burn" and that aroma.

Lonely is a funny thing. It's almost like another person. After a while it will keep you company if you let it.

—ANN PACKER

I came across this passage several years ago while listening to the audiobook of Ann Packer's novel *The Dive from Clausen's Pier*. I almost gasped when I heard it because it opened my heart and mind to a possibility I'd never considered. I've carried those few sentences in my heart ever since. I hope they bring you as much comfort as they've brought me. Her words have taught me not to resist loneliness and not to feel averse to it. Instead, I treat it as a familiar guest who shows up from time to time. I let it keep me company, knowing that it will eventually go on its way, making way for glorious (or at least bittersweet) solitude.

27

Healing Loneliness through Mindfulness

The worst loneliness is to not be comfortable
with yourself.

—MARK TWAIN

EARLY ON during my tenure as the dean of students at the law school, I discovered how nourishing mindfulness practice could be when I was alone.

With the best of intentions, people often wanted to do business over lunch. But I knew that even if I enjoyed their company, meeting in that way would still be work. Lunchtime was my only opportunity during the day to put aside the pressures of the job. So I told my assistant not to make appointments between 11:30 a.m. and 1:00 p.m. If someone asked to discuss business with me over lunch, I politely declined and arranged to meet him or her during non-lunch hours.

I found a nearby café that neither law students nor my colleagues frequented, and I began a daily outing. Except on days when a noon event kept me at the law school, I left the building at 11:30

a.m. I'd find the dirt path through the campus arboretum that led to the café. I'd walk the path slowly and mindfully, paying careful attention to the physical sensation of each foot as it touched the ground, noticing the trees and bushes around me, listening to the birds, taking in nature's aromas.

For the six years I was in the dean's office, I took this same path. I bought an oversized umbrella and rain boots so I could go on my jaunt in the pouring rain and the blustery wind—much to the dismay of some of the office staff! My awareness of impermanence was heightened because, with mindfulness as my guide, the walk was different every time. I could see the changing seasons on display in the plants and wildlife around me.

Seeing me from a distance, the café workers would have my espresso drink ready by the time I got to the door. Once inside, I continued my mindfulness practice by "letting the world speak for itself," to borrow a phrase from Pema Chödrön. I didn't read or think about work. I just sat and ate, watching the hustle and bustle of café life at lunchtime. Then I walked back to the law school along the same dirt path. I'd return to work relaxed and rejuvenated from what I came to think of as my daily mindfulness outing. I was alone, but I never felt lonely.

From "alone" to "lonely."

Being alone is a neutral state. It's just the fact of being by yourself. By contrast, loneliness is a painful emotional state, often accompanied by feelings of rejection, sadness, and self-blame. When illness forced me to leave work and take up residence in my bedroom, suddenly, I didn't like being alone—at all. Now I wasn't just alone; I was lonely. And it was the "worst loneliness," to which Mark Twain refers, because I wasn't comfortable with myself anymore.

I didn't feel rejected, but I was terribly sad and plagued by self-blame. I was convinced that my loneliness was proof of some character flaw. It took me several years to stop judging myself negatively for feeling as I did. Only then could I begin to bring caring attention to the loneliness. I started by giving up my resistance to it. In other words, I made room for it in my heart, even though it was an unpleasant feeling. Without blaming myself for its presence, I simply noticed how loneliness felt, including the sadness that accompanied it. To my surprise, when I allowed myself to feel the pain, the loneliness lost its tight-fisted grip on me. This gave me some breathing room and, in that space, I could begin to take a closer look at this emotion.

Bringing mindfulness to loneliness.

It's not uncommon for people to suffer from loneliness. Those who work around other people can feel lonely in their presence. Others may have loneliness descend on them as soon as they get home. If you're not a stranger to this painful emotion, becoming familiar with how it operates in your life can help you address it skillfully.

Before you begin to investigate loneliness, try to let go of any feelings of self-blame. A good way to do this is to remind yourself that everyone gets lonely at times. It's not a sign of weakness. It's just a mental state that's arisen due to conditions in your life.

Once you've accepted the feeling of loneliness—enough that you feel comfortable in its presence—you can begin to examine it by asking yourself some questions. Do certain experiences trigger it, like talking to others about their plans? Is it worse on certain days or at certain times of the day? How much is the loneliness the result of your desire to be with others, and how much is due to your not feeling comfortable with your own company?

You can continue this investigation by asking if you're telling yourself exaggerated and distorted stories, such as "I'll always be lonely" or "No one else I know is lonely." The former is highly unlikely to be true. As for the latter, how would you know? We rarely know the inner life of other people.

Becoming mindful in this way of what factors give rise to loneliness in your life, and learning to question the validity of the stories you tell yourself about it, makes it more manageable.

Then, with an attitude of kind benevolence toward yourself, let the loneliness be and allow compassion to arise over any suffering you're experiencing. Find just the right words by drawing on what your investigation has revealed to you about the loneliness you're feeling. Silently or softly, repeat phrases such as "It's hard to be by myself after hearing about everyone else's plans"; "It's painful to be alone on the weekends"; "It's not my fault that I'm lonely."

As you say these words, you might stroke one arm with the hand of the other. I do this often as a way to deepen self-compassion. Gently hold the loneliness in mindful awareness in this way, while at the same time also maintaining awareness that, like all mental states, loneliness is subject to change and so is not a permanent feature of who you are.

Alone in my bedroom, practicing mindfulness in this way, I gradually made peace with loneliness. Recall from chapter 23 the words of Thich Nhat Hanh: "Awareness is like the sun. When it shines on things, they are transformed." Sure enough, over time, the loneliness I was feeling transformed from a painful mental state to the neutral fact of being by myself. This opened the door for me to explore ways in which being alone might enrich my life.

Being alone heightens my awareness of the world around me.

Through mindfulness, I rediscovered what I'd known during those lunchtime outings: when I'm by myself, my powers of observation are more keen. In a passage from *Emma*, Jane Austen said this about Emma as she looked out her window at the small happenings in the village street below: "A mind lively and at ease, can do

with seeing nothing, and can see nothing that does not answer."
I've learned to do with seeing and hearing beauty in the small happenings in my bedroom: a spider, dropping from the ceiling on a silken thread, only to stop a foot above the bed; a fly, dashing around the bedroom like some crazy freeway driver; the sound of the starlings in the elm tree right outside the bedroom window.

The spiritual teacher Ram Dass said, "The quieter you become, the more you can hear." I was reminded of these words when a woman wrote to me saying that illness had forced her to trade a life of activity for one of stillness, but that when she uses that stillness to observe her small world closely, "it almost seems like an even trade."

Being alone gets my creative juices flowing.

"I dwell in possibility," wrote Emily Dickinson. I've discovered that being alone opens possibilities in my mind because it facilitates what I think of as creative daydreaming. My mind wanders freely, allowing ideas to come and go until something becomes the seed for the next piece of writing or a new crochet project.

In addition, although I'm not a poet by any means, I've discovered that writing short poems when I'm alone is a satisfying creative outlet. I include this one just to give you an idea of what you can do:

> Hot summer sun
> coming through the window.
> Please don't melt my laptop!

I wrote it one morning when I forgot to put the shades down in my bedroom and noticed that the summer sun was shining directly on my computer. I put my hand on the keyboard, and it was very hot. I experienced a momentary scare (after all, my laptop is where I do all my writing!). Then, I put the shade down, sat back on my bed, and wrote this poem.

Being alone allows me to dictate the rhythm of the day.

When I'm alone, I live at my own rhythm. Some people do better with a fixed schedule, but, for me, since I never know how I'm going to feel physically at any particular time on any given day, not having a set timetable is beneficial to both my mind and body. I might eat dinner for lunch or breakfast for dinner. And, of course, there's no set time to engage in creative daydreaming. As an added bonus, when I'm doing something because it best fits the rhythm of my day, I've discovered that I do it with more intention, which means I'm giving more careful attention to the present moment.

Being alone makes me more attentive to others when I'm not alone.

Since I've been isolated by illness, when I do see people I care about, I'm much more aware of everything about them—from their outer appearance, to what it is I enjoy about their company, to what might be troubling them. I think I'm a better friend. I'm more attentive to strangers, too. People watching has become a challenging practice—to observe without letting on that I'm observing! In short, I feel as if I'm seeing friends and strangers afresh, with new eyes.

Being alone opens the door to spiritual exploration.

Being alone offers the opportunity to nurture the inner life, whether through prayer or meditation or cultivating compassion for all beings. In the quiet space of isolation from the world outside, we can reflect on life, including its wonders and its mysteries.

In some sense, all of us are alone, because no one experiences our lives for us and no one encounters our particular mixture of joys and sorrows. Reflecting on this can help us appreciate the uniqueness of the life that each of us has.

And yet, although in some sense we are all alone, we are also interconnected and interdependent with everything and everyone around us, from the air we breath, to the food we eat, from the people we're close to, to the people we'll never meet but who affect our lives every day. My spiritual exploration often takes the form of a practice called *tonglen* because it heightens my awareness of this interconnectedness of all life.

Tonglen is a unique Tibetan compassion practice. In many meditation practices, we're instructed to breathe in peaceful and healing thoughts and images and to breathe out any suffering we're feeling. By contrast, in tonglen, we do the opposite—we breathe in the suffering of others, and then as we breathe out, we offer whatever measure of kindness, compassion, and peace of mind we have to give, even the slightest bit.

I practice tonglen when I'm alone to help me feel connected to people, no matter what their circumstances and no matter where they live on the planet. I call to mind people whose lives, on the surface, seem so different from mine—a poverty-stricken family in a third-world country, a single mother of three in a crime-ridden neighborhood in the US, people living in war zones. As I picture them in their environment, I breathe their suffering into my heart. Then, on the out-breath, I release that suffering and offer to them whatever kindness, compassion, and peace of mind I have to give at the moment.

Tonglen makes me acutely aware that, although everyone's life is a unique mix of joys and sorrows, we are more alike than we are different. We all experience difficulties and we all share the same hopes and dreams for ourselves and our loved ones.

I hope you'll try tonglen. If you're not comfortable breathing in other people's suffering, just breathe normally and call to mind the people with whom you wish to connect. Then, in whatever way feels natural to you, send them thoughts of kindness and compassion. You need not breathe in others' suffering in order to feel connected to them.

I still feel lonely at times. When this happens, I don't resist it. I regard it as a familiar guest who wasn't invited but still shows up periodically, making itself at home for a while. Using mindfulness practice, I acknowledge the loneliness, hold it gently in my awareness, and treat myself with compassion for any sadness I'm experiencing.

Zen teacher Dainin Katagiri said, "One can be lonely and not be tossed away by it." And so I open my heart to the loneliness and let it be, knowing that the sweetness of being alone without feeling lonely is waiting in the wings.

28

Coping with Isolation During Holidays and Other Gatherings

> *The heart that breaks open can contain*
> *the whole universe.*
>
> —JOANNA MACY

ONE OF THE toughest challenges of being chronically ill is the necessity of adjusting to a different way of spending holidays and other special gatherings, such as weddings. After I became chronically ill, the activities that had once brought me the greatest joy suddenly became the very activities that exacerbated my symptoms. Special gatherings are among those events.

We want to contribute fully to the festivities—helping with the planning, the cooking, and even the cleanup. On the other hand, we also know that even limited participation is likely to trigger a flare of symptoms that will result in "payback" later. In addition, many people who are chronically ill have compromised immune systems, making it hard for them to fight infections. Close gatherings, especially during the winter months, increase the risk of catching a cold or the flu. This can leave a person bedbound for weeks or months and, in some cases, hospitalized.

I've had to accept that most holidays and other special gatherings are out of reach for me now. However, one of them—Thanksgiving—I do my best to still celebrate with others. On Thanksgiving, our son Jamal and his family, my brother-in-law and sister-in-law, and a couple of close friends come for a feast that my husband cooks. Invariably, when everyone arrives, I start out with a burst of energetic socializing. I wasn't this way before I got sick, so I'm positive this is a reaction to the amount of time I spend alone. It's as if I'm in a panic to get in everything I want to tell everyone before, like Cinderella, my time is up.

I'm sure I'd be able to stay at the gathering longer if I paced myself. To this end, I always give myself a little lecture before everyone arrives: "Breathe deeply, move slowly, and don't chat up a storm." I've yet to be able to stick to my plan; once I join the festivities, it's too hard to half-participate. As a result, I overdo it until I feel as if I'm about to drop unless I lie down. Imagine having the flu when people come over for Thanksgiving. You'd only last so long before you'd have no choice but to excuse yourself.

And so inevitably the time comes when I have to leave the gathering and retreat to the bedroom. Sometimes I'm prompted by my husband who watches out for me, even when I'm not watching out for myself. (See chapter 1, where I suggest that everyone try to find such an ally.)

Once in my bedroom, I face the toughest challenge: coping with the sadness and sorrow I feel at being isolated from others. One reason it's a challenge is that my "retreat" tends to coincide with the time when socializing has become easygoing and mellow. When people first arrive at a gathering, it's not unusual for the conversation to be polite and guarded for a while—except for little "burst of energy" me, of course! But after a few hours and some good food and drink, everyone is relaxed. By the time I'm forced to excuse myself, I retire to the sounds of warm conversation, spiced with peals of laughter. It's the very moment I want to be with everyone.

When I get to my bedroom, I always think, "If only the gathering were starting *right now*, I could be there for the best part." This reflection used to be accompanied by quiet sobbing—quiet, so no one would hear me. Over the years, though, I've come up with some techniques to help ease the sadness and sorrow that arise when I'm forced to isolate myself from others. I hope they're helpful to you.

No blame!

As I've noted in earlier chapters, self-blame is a common reaction to becoming chronically ill. You may think it's your fault that you're sick or in pain. You may blame yourself for having to skip a gathering or leave it early. Or you may feel as if you're not doing your fair share to contribute to the festivities.

This last source of negative self-judgment—the feeling of not carrying my weight—can still pop up for me at Thanksgiving. My husband does the shopping and the cooking. Everyone who comes brings more food, and my son and daughter-in-law set the table and do the dishes afterward. I consider it a major accomplishment when I'm able to contribute a pumpkin pie, although even with this relatively simple task I've had to make adjustments; my favorite part of pie-making was always preparing the crust, and I've reluctantly had to let that go. No one seems to mind that it's a store-bought crust, but I secretly feel that my pie is not the real deal. That's a bit of "no blame" I'm still working on.

Learning not to judge myself negatively for becoming chronically ill has been a tremendous relief. Even more, the realization that I can be the way I am without blame has brought with it a newfound sense of freedom. For all of us, the reward for setting aside self-blame is that we can begin to treat ourselves with compassion. Self-blame and self-compassion are incompatible. I hope that all of you who are chronically ill will make the commitment to replace the former with the latter.

Practice self-compassion.

When being isolated makes me sad, I don't resist it. Resisting painful emotions tends to strengthen them. So the first thing I do is to gently acknowledge that sadness is present. Next, I think of specific words that address, with compassion, how I'm feeling at the moment; then I actually speak those words to myself.

I hope you'll try this. Pick some phrases that fit your particular circumstance and repeat them silently or softly to yourself: "It's so hard to leave the holiday gathering right when the conversation was getting good" or "I'm so sad to be alone in the bedroom." Repeat your phrases, perhaps while stroking one arm with the hand of the other. Stroking my arm or my cheek with my hand never fails to ease my emotional pain.

If speaking to yourself in this way brings tears to your eyes, that's okay. They're tears of compassion. To quote Lord Byron, "The dew of compassion is a tear."

Cultivate joy for others.

I also work on feeling joy for those who are still gathering together. I think about the good time everyone is having and try to feel happy for them. Buddhists call this *mudita*—feeling joy for other people who are happy. Initially, when you try to feel joy for others, it's not unusual for envy to pop into your mind instead. This is a perfectly understandable reaction to having to miss out on so much. If this happens to you, remember, *no blame*! Simply acknowledge with compassion that you're feeling envious, and when you're ready, try again.

When I practice feeling joy for other people, it helps if I picture their smiling faces and (unless I'm hearing it "live" from my bedroom) imagine the sound of their good-hearted conversation and laughter. Eventually, even though I may still be sad, I'm also able to feel happy for them. And once in a while, something special happens: I begin to feel joy myself, as if everyone is having a good time *for* me.

Stick to describing your emotions in a neutral fashion.

In chapter 11, "Mindfulness Practices That Address Physical Discomfort," I described a practice that I adapted from Byron Katie in which you ground yourself in the present moment by neutrally describing what's happening in your life right now.

This mindfulness practice is also helpful when feelings of sadness and sorrow accompany being alone. Describing isolation in a neutral fashion can keep those painful emotions from intensifying, and it also serves as a reminder that what you're feeling is a temporary mental state; these emotions have arisen and they will pass.

To try this practice, the next time isolation triggers mental suffering for you, describe the experience of being alone without using emotionally charged words. Instead of saying "Lying on the bed, feeling *unbearably* isolated," simply say "Lying on the bed, feeling isolated." Words like "unbearably," "dismally," "intolerably," and "miserably" add an emotional punch that's likely to intensify the mental suffering you're experiencing.

In addition, these emotionally charged words can lead you to start spinning stressful stories, such as "I'll be left out of things for the rest of my life" or "No one cares that I'm in the bedroom by myself." These stories—which we tell ourselves and then believe without question—only make matters worse. There's no rational reason to believe you'll be left out of things for the rest of your life or that no one cares about you. The sadness and sorrow you're experiencing are not built-in, permanent features of who you are. They're just what you happen to be feeling at this moment.

This practice may require you to change your habitual way of talking to yourself, but learning to describe your present-moment experience in a neutral way enables you to hold more lightly any emotional pain that accompanies being isolated. Then, treating yourself with compassion, you can wait until the painful feeling passes out of your mind.

Practice tonglen.

As I described in the previous chapter, tonglen is a powerful way to feel connected to others; this helps ease the emotional pain that often accompanies isolation. You can begin by breathing in the suffering of others. Then, on the out-breath, breathe out whatever measure of kindness, compassion, and peace of mind you have to offer them, even if it's just a little bit.

I didn't discover the healing power of tonglen until I'd been chronically ill for six years. Refusing to accept that I was too sick to throw a welcoming party when my granddaughter Cam was born, I made all the arrangements from my bed. But when the day arrived, I was too sick to attend. After I broke the news to my son over the phone, I hung up and began sobbing.

After about ten minutes, I suddenly realized that there were people all over the world who, like me, were too sick or in too much pain—or both—to be able to attend a special gathering. I began to picture these people in my mind, as vividly as possible. Then I breathed in their sadness and sorrow, and I breathed out whatever kindness, compassion, and peace of mind I had to give them.

As I did this, I became aware that I was breathing in my own sadness and sorrow, and that when I breathed out kindness, com-passion, and peace of mind for them, I was also sending these sentiments to myself. I realized that tonglen was a two-for-one compassion practice: I wasn't just cultivating kindness, compas-sion, and peace for others for whom isolation was painful; I was cultivating it for myself.

I encourage you to try this the next time that being isolated due to limitations imposed by your health leaves you feeling sad and sorrowful. Remember that if you find it difficult to breathe in other people's suffering, modify the practice. Rather than taking in their suffering on the in-breath, breathe normally and call to mind others who, like you, are suffering emotionally from being isolated. Then, in whatever way feels comfortable to you, send them thoughts of kindness, compassion, and peace of mind.

I love the effect that this practice has on the unpleasant feeling that I'm missing out on everything. When I practice tonglen, any mental suffering that isolation has triggered becomes manageable because I feel deeply connected to others who are feeling the same way. As eco-philosopher Joanna Macy said in the epigraph that begins this chapter, "The heart that breaks open can contain the whole universe."

VI. Enjoy the Life You Have

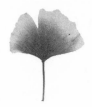

29

Beware of "Good Old Days Syndrome"

Remembrance of things past is not necessarily
the remembrance of things as they were.

—MARCEL PROUST

OR THE MOST part, I've adjusted to my new life but, occasionally, I still catch myself engaged in distorted thinking about the past. I've taken to calling it "Good Old Days Syndrome."

When it attacks, I put my pre-illness life on a pedestal. My thinking runs along these lines: "Before I got sick, everything was perfect: working at the law school was always a pleasure; my family life was ideal; I was free to go wherever I wanted, whenever I wanted."

True, true, and true? Not exactly. Being a law professor was not always enjoyable. Workloads could be demanding; reading exams and papers could be sheer drudgery. And although I enjoyed most of the students, occasionally one could make my life difficult. When I was the dean of students, one troubled student was the stuff of nightmares; for a brief time, I had to be given police protection.

My family life was definitely good, but it could be stressful at times. We had our share of conflicts and disagreements, some of them temporary, others ongoing.

And do I really believe that I could go anywhere I wanted to go at will?

No, life wasn't perfect before I got sick. It had its share of easy times and hard times, of getting my way and not getting my way. When I find myself idealizing that "old" life by convincing myself that I was always happy, I try to remember that this is a distorted view of the past that invariably leaves me feeling bad about the present.

We also tend to reminisce about other eras as if *they* were the Good Old Days. In his NBC newscast of April 8, 2013, Brian Williams began his report on the death of Annette Funicello by wistfully referring to the 1950s as "a sweeter era, one of genuine innocence." I don't think so. Not only was that the era of Red baiting, but in those "sweet and innocent" 1950s, in many places in the US, it would have been a crime for my two children to marry the people they fell in love with—simply because those two people happen to be of different races than my children.

My Good Old Days era is the '60s. Ah, those were the days: rock and roll, flower power, love love love. And yet those were also the days of the civil rights struggle and its associated atrocities. I once saw a documentary about Birmingham, Alabama, in 1963; police used hoses and police dogs to stop children from peacefully marching to protest segregation. (The children had to march by themselves because their parents had been told they'd lose their jobs if they participated even during off-work hours.) The footage in the story showed children being bitten by police dogs and knocked to the ground by high-powered hoses.

And then there were earlier eras when people died of diseases that we're now protected against by popping a pill or getting a vaccination. A family friend who grew up in the 1930s once told me that at the first sign of sniffles in the winter, her parents wouldn't let her play outside until spring. They didn't want to take a chance that the sniffles would turn into bronchitis or some other kind of bacterial infection, for which, today, we'd just take an antibiotic.

Try this test. The following passage was written by a well-known author. Take a guess at when she wrote it:

> We are so overwhelmed with things these days that our lives are all, more or less, cluttered... Everyone is hurrying and usually just a little late. Notice the faces of the people who rush past on the streets... They nearly all have a strained, harassed look, and anyone you meet will tell you there is no time for anything anymore.

What's your guess? 2015? 1990? Whenever you were growing up? Does it have you waxing nostalgic about the Good Old Days when life was slower-paced and much more quiet?

Test over: It was written in 1924 by Laura Ingalls Wilder—while living on a farm in rural Missouri!

Here's an account of a recent attack of Good Old Days Syndrome. My husband was out of town, so I had to go to the pharmacy on my own to refill a prescription. I ran into a friend whom I hadn't seen for about ten years. We embraced and found a place to sit and then chatted for about fifteen minutes, catching up on news about our families and our mutual friends.

After we parted, I was overcome with sadness and fell into a funk over this lost friendship, which I was suddenly cherishing deeply. As I do when I recognize that I'm dissatisfied and unhappy, I looked for the source of my misery in some kind of frustrated desire. I traced the feeling until I found that place where I wasn't getting what I wanted. And there it was: I wanted this friendship to be as wonderful as it once had been.

Then it dawned on me; this friendship had never been the way I was fantasizing it to have been in the Good Old Days. She and I were never truly close. We mostly saw each other because we had a few friends in common. We liked each other well enough, but neither of us was motivated to build a close relationship. And yet there I was, mocking up a distorted memory of the Good Old Days—and then feeling miserable about it.

As soon as I became aware of this distorted thinking, my funk lifted. Yes, I was still a bit blue, but it was a sadness that periodically arises over my isolation and lack of contact with the many people I used to hang out with. I know this sadness well; it comes and goes. I can ease its pain by being extra kind to myself. This "comes and goes" sadness is an entirely different feeling from the miserable mood I'd fallen into from having romanticized a Good Old Days relationship with this woman, when that relationship had, in fact, never existed.

So be on alert for Good Old Days Syndrome and remember that life has its ups and downs, its joys and sorrows, its justices and injustices, in every era and in every decade.

30

Why *Not* Me?

Freedom is instantaneous the moment we accept
the way things are.

—KAREN MAEZEN MILLER

A WELL-KNOWN BUDDHIST story known as the Mustard Seed helped me learn that continually asking "Why Me?" was an unrealistic assessment of the human condition that had become an ongoing source of suffering for me.

In the Mustard Seed story, Kisa Gotami was a young mother who refused to believe that her young son had died. She carried him door-to-door in her village, pleading for medicine. People told her that it was too late for medicine, but she was unable to understand or accept that. Then someone suggested that she ask the Buddha for medicine. When she did, he told her to bring him a mustard seed from a house that had never experienced death.

She began going door-to-door again, this time telling people that the Buddha needed a mustard seed to make medicine for her son. No one refused her request. But when she asked, "Has this house experienced death?" the response was always, "Yes, of course," and so she'd leave empty-handed.

After some time, she realized that impermanence and death were universal. She buried her son and returned to the Buddha. When he asked if she had obtained the mustard seed, she said: "Finished is the matter of the mustard seed. You have restored me."

This may seem like a harsh tale, but I appreciate how the Buddha knew that the best way for Kisa Gotami to make peace with one of life's harsh realities was to touch that reality firsthand, rather than listen to a lecture from him.

Whenever I hear the Mustard Seed story, I think about how I've responded to traumatic events in my own life. Like everyone else, my life has had its share of sorrows—some of them deep sorrows. My father's death when I was ten years old is at the top of the list. Becoming chronically ill in 2001 is near the top.

My father and I were extremely close; his death was devastating to me. I remember looking at other kids my age and asking "Why me?" over and over again, in an achingly painful refrain. I was angry at the world and (it's hard to admit) angry at my father for dying. Unfortunately, no one in my life had the skill to tell me a child's version of the Mustard Seed—a tale that could have gently communicated to me that life is unpredictable and can feel horribly unfair but that, with time, I'd be able to accept what happened and begin to enjoy life again.

Many decades later, when I got sick and didn't recover, the "Why me?" refrain started up again. I blamed myself for losing my career and for having to give up so many activities that I loved. I felt unfairly treated by the world and by my body. But repeatedly asking "Why me?" served only to intensify the resentment I was feeling and the blame I was directing at myself.

After several years, I finally began to change my response to being chronically ill. Remembering the Mustard Seed story helped;

it enabled me to accept that all people face unexpected upheavals in their lives. This meant that my "Why me?" refrain—which left me feeling as if I'd been singled out in some way—was a distorted view of the human condition.

I was also helped by the writings of Zen teacher Charlotte Joko Beck. In her book *Everyday Zen*, she writes:

> Our life is always all right. There's nothing wrong with it. Even if we have horrendous problems, it's just our life.

This passage was transformative for me. "Why me?" became irrelevant when I realized that my life was just my life, that it was all right, even though it included giving up a career years before I felt ready, feeling sick every day, and being severely restricted in my activities. *It's just my life.* The realization that there was nothing wrong with my life was a tremendous relief because it meant there was nothing wrong *with me.*

I was also helped by country music artist Rosanne Cash. In October 2009, she was a guest on NPR's *Fresh Air*. Cash had put her career on hold because she had to have brain surgery for a rare but benign condition. The host, Terry Gross, asked her if she ever found herself asking "Why me?" Cash replied "no"—that, in fact, she found herself saying "Why *not* me?" since she had health insurance, a career she could keep despite the need for a long recuperation, and a spouse who was a wonderful caregiver.

I know that not everyone is fortunate in the ways that Rosanne Cash mentioned. For many people, stress over money and lack of support are ongoing challenges. And yet, remember Kisa Gotami and the mustard seed; no one gets a pass on life's difficulties. Not even Ms. Cash—think about the stress and the fear she must have experienced before and after her brain surgery, with its risks and uncertain outcome. Rosanne Cash's "Why *not* me?" drives home to me the reality that life is not necessarily fair, even though as children, we're taught that it should be.

Odd as it may sound, the day I realized that life is not fair, I felt a burden lift off my shoulders because, at last, I could give up the exhausting but fruitless battle to *make* it fair. It's been such a relief that I now count the expression "Life isn't fair" among my equanimity practices. When I don't expect life to be fair, I'm open to the way it actually is at the moment, including the unexpected turns it takes along the way—even the sorrowful turns.

As Joko Beck suggests, there's nothing wrong with us when the going gets rough. Even when our expectations are turned upside down, it's just how life is for us. This perspective helps us rest in the accepting calm of equanimity. It also opens the door for self-compassion to arise because, instead of turning away in aversion from our struggles, we open our hearts to whatever life is serving up at the moment.

Inspired by an ancient Buddhist story, a contemporary Zen teacher, and a country music artist, when I start to sink into that "Why me?" way of thinking, whether it be over the "unfair" turn my health took in 2001 or over any disappointment or sorrow, I know I'll feel more at peace and enjoy life more if, in a kind and gentle voice, I turn "Why me?" into "Why *not* me?"

31

Don't Let Envy and Resentment Keep You from Enjoying the Life You Have

Human happiness is a disposition of mind and
not a condition of circumstances.

—JOHN LOCKE

WHEN I WAS twelve, I discovered paradise—a chain of islands halfway across the Pacific Ocean from my Los Angeles home. *Hawaii.* It was a difficult time in my life. My father had died two years before. Losing him was a shock, and I still missed him terribly. I was entering my teenage years as a sullen and self-conscious kid. Then my mother took me and my brother to Hawaii, and I was happy for the first time since I'd lost my father.

Seeing the difference in me, she took us to the islands three summers in a row. I loved the tropical climate. I loved the fragrant air. I loved the music. And I loved to surf. When I was riding a wave, that sullen teenager felt carefree and happy.

As an adult with a young family, I couldn't afford to go to

Hawaii. However, I needed only to hear Hawaiian music to feel transported back to paradise, always with the thought "Some day, some day."

As soon as we could afford vacations, I whisked the family off to Hawaii. From then on, my husband and I went almost every summer, first with our children and then, after they'd grown, just the two of us. We explored every island that allowed visitors. In 1995, I found the hideaway on Molokai that I wrote about in chapter 2. We returned to it year after year.

When I became chronically ill in 2001, abruptly, the trips stopped. I haven't been able to travel since. For many years, I was angry at my body—as if I'd been wronged by it because it was keeping me from doing what I wanted to do. That Want Monster from chapter 5 was whispering *loudly* in my ear! But I could not get my way.

I've worked hard to make peace with this unexpected change in my life plans. For the most part, my suffering over not being able to travel has given way to an appreciation for the life I do have, altered though it is.

Then one day in 2012, my close friend Kari told me that she and her family were about to leave for a two-week vacation in Hawaii. I felt a rush of sadness but it passed quickly, giving way to that joyful state of mudita that I wrote about in chapter 28. I felt genuinely happy for my friend. "Be sure to post pictures!" I told her enthusiastically.

But when she uploaded that first picture—a beach on Kauai—I drew back from it physically and mentally, and this turned out not to be a momentary reaction. I couldn't bring myself to look at any of the pictures she was posting, and I became agitated and irritable. "I was so happy for Kari. What's going on with me?" I wondered.

It didn't take long to realize that I was envious that Kari was in Hawaii and I was not. Even more, I felt a touch of resentment. Envy arises when we want what someone else has. Resentment is also present if we believe we're not getting it because of some perceived unfairness or injustice in the world or on the part of another person. My wanting to have the Hawaii experience that Kari was having is an example of envy. The bitter feeling that it wasn't fair that she got to go and I didn't is an example of resentment.

Given the struggles we face individually and globally, this incident with Kari may seem trivial: a friend was in Hawaii, and I was envious and resentful. Big deal. And yet when stressful emotions take hold of us, even over a minor matter such as a trip we can't take, they can be so compelling and overpowering that they impair our ability to function effectively in life.

This is exactly what was happening to me as I grew more and more upset about Kari's trip, even though I knew it was insignificant in the big scheme of things. What could I do to ease the suffering I was experiencing? I decided to look at envy and resentment through the lens of the four-step approach I introduced in chapter 8, "The Many Benefits of Patience." Again, here are the four steps:

- ► Recognize it.
- ► Label it.
- ► Investigate it.
- ► Let it be.

Although I'll use the "Hawaii incident" as an example, I encourage you to explore this practice by bringing to mind something in your life about which you're feeling envy or resentment, or both. It could be related solely to your health, but it could also be a friend who's in a new romantic relationship, a coworker who got a promotion, a family member who's rolling in cash, or an acquaintance who always seems carefree and happy. As you read what follows, try applying the four steps to your specific situation.

Recognize it.

It may seem as if recognizing the presence of a stressful emotion would be easy, but it can be a challenge. One reason is that we can be so focused on the *object* of whatever emotions are present that we mistakenly believe that the unease we're experiencing is caused by that object. In my situation, I was so focused on the object of my envy and resentment—Kari being in Hawaii instead of me—that when I saw her photo of Kauai, I thought the photo itself was the source of my unhappiness. It wasn't until I pointedly asked myself "What am I feeling?" and "What emotions are present?" that I recognized that the suffering I was experiencing wasn't being imposed on me from the outside but was in my own mind in the form of envy and resentment.

Another reason it took me a while to recognize that envy and resentment were present is that I love Kari; this kept me from seeing that she could still be a trigger for painful emotions on my part. As Buddhist teacher Jack Kornfield likes to say, "The mind has no shame." In my experience, he's right. The mind is going to think and feel what it's going to think and feel, even if we wish it wouldn't!

Recognizing the presence of a stressful emotion is a mindfulness skill. It requires paying caring attention to what we're feeling. Caring attention is *attention without judgment*, which includes not judging our "shameless" minds. If we're busy blaming ourselves for being unhappy, it becomes virtually impossible to unearth the stressful emotions that lie beneath that unhappiness—in this case, envy and resentment.

Label it.

The purpose of labeling an emotion is to hold it in awareness so that we can investigate it. Once again, a nonjudgmental attitude is essential. Stressful emotions can be fertile ground for judging ourselves negatively. Many of us think we shouldn't feel certain emotions because they aren't appropriate and reflect poorly on us. However, everyone experiences his or her share of unpleasant and painful emotions.

As soon as I realized that envy and resentment had arisen over Kari's trip, my inner critic was ready to pounce. I immediately started judging myself negatively for feeling this way about someone for whom I care deeply. As if envy and resentment weren't unpleasant enough, now I'd added another layer of suffering in the form of blaming myself for feeling these two emotions in the first place. It was only through nonjudgmental labeling that I was able to quiet the inner critic.

The best way to label an emotion nonjudgmentally is to regard it as an uninvited guest. Think of it this way: you didn't invite it over, yet neither will you push the door closed in its face. The Buddha often used the phrase "I see you" to label a mental state. I picture him saying it in a friendly, even teasing, tone. Here's how I labeled the emotions I was feeling about Kari's trip:

- ▸ My old friend envy has arisen.
- ▸ Feeling resentment too.
- ▸ I see you, envy and resentment.

Investigate it.

Investigating a stressful emotion keeps it from intensifying because it's no longer just sitting in our minds, brewing.

Holding the envy and resentment without judgment in my

awareness, I started investigating them by paying attention to how they felt in my body. Pleasant? Unpleasant? Definitely the latter. I could even feel some muscles contracting. I also noticed that I was breathing more shallowly than usual. I took a deep breath and made a conscious effort to relax my body. That alone eased my distress a bit.

Then I looked at my mind. When I'm suffering due to a painful emotion, I can almost always trace it back to an unfulfilled longing or desire. Here, the desire wasn't hard to pinpoint: I wanted to go to Hawaii, and this wanting was more than a preference. My longing to go was so strong that I was experiencing it as a need: "I *need* to go to Hawaii," I was telling myself. No wonder I was miserable!

Further investigation revealed that I'd been linking going to Hawaii with my very ability to be happy. This had me spinning an unrealistic story that was intensifying the envy and resentment: "I need to go to Hawaii in order to feel happy again." Absurd as this may sound, I'd convinced myself that this was true. Like most people, I'd been conditioned from childhood to believe that getting what I wanted in life would bring me sustained and lasting happiness.

I've worked hard to undo this harmful conditioning. Even so, I can still fall prey to it when an intense desire clouds my ability to see that minds are as changeable as everything else in the world. What we want today isn't necessarily what we'll want tomorrow. A desire fulfilled soon gives way to a new desire—going to Tahiti perhaps? Reflecting on this helped me see the absurdity of believing that going to Hawaii would solve all my problems.

My investigation also revealed that the envy and resentment had me feeling possessive about Hawaii. If I couldn't go there, I didn't want anyone else to either. This generated another stressful story:

"It's *my* Hawaii. Kari and her family are in *my* Hawaii." I know that sounds childish, but it's what was going on in my mind. When I became aware of this possessiveness, a slight smile came to my face, and I shook my head at the mind's seemingly infinite ability to derail our attempts to be at peace with our lives, however that life is unfolding at the moment.

Further investigation finally allowed me to shed light on the source of my resentment. Recall that resentment is the bitter feeling that arises when we believe we're not getting what we want because we think we've been treated unfairly by someone or something. I didn't feel unfairly treated by Kari, but I did feel unfairly treated by life. This gave rise to a third stressful story: "It's not fair that I'm sick and can't go where I want to, when I want to."

Bringing into conscious awareness the stories that are triggered by stressful emotions makes it possible to examine the faulty assumptions that underlie those stories. When I questioned the validity of my three stories, I saw that none of them had any basis in fact:

- ▸ "I need to go to Hawaii in order to feel happy again."—Not true.
- ▸ "Kari and her family are in *my* Hawaii."—I don't own Hawaii!
- ▸ "It's not fair that I'm sick."—All bodies are subject to illness at one time or another in life.

The insights gained from investigating a stressful emotion—noticing how it feels physically, looking for the desire that underlies it, questioning the validity of the stories we tell ourselves about it—is likely to have already weakened its tight-fisted grip on us. Then we can move on to the next step.

Let it be.

When we command ourselves to let go of a painful emotion, we open ourselves to self-blame if we fail in our efforts. In addition, the emotion may actually intensify because we're adding aversion to what we're feeling. So rather than trying to push an unpleasant emotion out of our minds by telling ourselves "Let it go, let it go," I suggest the more compassionate "Let it be."

To let envy and resentment be, it helps to reflect on how they're not built-in qualities of who we are. There's no reason to take on the identity of "I'm an envious person" or "I'm a resentful person." Envy and resentment are simply emotions that have momentarily arisen as a result of past and current conditions in our lives.

Reflecting on my past conditioning, I realized that the envy and resentment I was feeling stemmed from the strong affection I'd developed for Hawaii at a time in my life when I was particularly vulnerable and needy. Remembering how unhappy I was after my father died became the catalyst for evoking compassion for myself.

Cultivating compassion is the kindest and most skillful way to *let it be*, no matter what stressful or painful emotion we're experiencing. I recommend silently or softly speaking kindly to yourself by finding words that specifically address your suffering. Here's how I spoke to myself with compassion: "It's hard not to be able to go to Hawaii when it's such a special place for me"; "I'm sad that I can't feel happy for Kari at this moment." Speaking in this way eased my suffering because it gave me permission to be present for how I was feeling.

As self-compassion deepens, the door to equanimity opens. A mind that is equanimous engages the full range of human emotions without negative self-judgment and with an even temper and a peaceful heart, knowing that, like all mental states, emotions are subject to the law of impermanence.

Wrapped in a cloak of compassion and steadied by equanimity, I patiently waited. Sure enough, the envy and resentment eventually weakened and passed out of my mind, leaving me feeling happy again for my friend and free to look for ways to enjoy life despite my limitations. Yes, it's true that I can no longer travel to my paradise, but as Tibetan Buddhist teacher Pema Chödrön so wisely reminds us: "It isn't the things that happen to us in our lives that cause us to suffer. It's how we relate to the things that happen to us that causes us to suffer."

It takes practice to learn to work skillfully with envy and resentment—or with any painful emotion. Be content to take baby steps. When you first try this four-step approach, don't be discouraged if you sometimes get lost or it feels like a muddle to you. Just take a deep breath and try again. We can go from suffering to not-suffering over and over again, so be patient. Patience is an act of self-compassion, and I hope you'll undertake this four-step approach in that spirit.

32

Slow Down and Savor Life

Climb Mount Fuji,
O snail,
but slowly, slowly.

—ISSA

IN THE EARLY 1990s, I discovered the value of slowing down.

At the time, I drove an '85 Ford LTD, nicknamed the Big White Boat by my children and their friends. I never liked driving on the freeway, even though I had to do it a lot. I'd hang out in the middle lane except when I wanted to pass a car. Then I'd pull into the left lane to get around it.

One day, I found myself driving in the far right lane. I noticed that the feeling-tone of the freeway experience was different. I felt more relaxed and was enjoying the scenery around me. I discovered that if I stayed in that lane and stuck to the speed limit, I wouldn't have to worry about passing cars, because they were going as slowly as I was. And no one was riding my bumper, since it was acceptable to go the speed limit in the far right lane. From that day forward, when on the freeway, it was "life in the slow lane" for me—that is, until chronic illness took me off the road-ways for the most part.

It's just as well that I don't drive on freeways anymore, because my strategy would no longer work. Today, most people exceed the speed limit even in the slow lane. In addition, traffic has increased to the point that I'd have to constantly be dodging cars merging onto the freeway from onramps—and so even in the slow lane, I wouldn't have the opportunity to admire the scenery. But it was a great idea while it lasted.

Since becoming chronically ill, I've taken that "slow lane" mentality and consciously applied it to other activities. Doing so helps me become more aware of what I'm doing and of everything around me, so I can appreciate and enjoy each moment of my life as it is, illness included. Additionally, slowing down can ease my symptoms.

This chapter explores some ways to ease back on the metaphorical throttle.

Double the time you think it will take to complete a task.

Even before I became chronically ill, I rarely completed a task in the time I'd allotted for it. (There must be some obscure cosmic law at work here.) This used to be a source of irritation and stress in my life. My to-do list was always so long that whenever a particular task took longer than I'd anticipated, it increased the pressure I felt to get through the rest of the list by the end of the day. As a result, I'd pick up the pace and move even faster. Now that I'm sick, I can't pick up the pace. In fact, I need to slow down. And so I've resolved to double the time I think it will take to complete a task.

Here's an example of how this works. I have a raised asparagus fern bed outside my front door. Periodically, the ferns spill over onto the walkway and I need to cut them back. When I assess the task, I estimate it will take twenty minutes at most, so I double the allotted time. Forty minutes is longer than I can physically work at this task at one time, so I cut back half the ferns on one day and the other half on the next.

Sure, the box looks odd for twenty-four hours—like half of a buzz cut—but no one seems to notice. And the benefits for me are well-worth it; I spare myself an exacerbation of symptoms, and by going more slowly and spreading the job over two days, I truly enjoy it—not once, but twice!

Become mindful of when you're multitasking and try to limit yourself to one activity.

Zen teachers like to say, "When eating, only eat. When resting, only rest. When thinking, only think." If you're like me, you may have such a strong multitasking habit that you're often not even aware that you're engaged in multiple tasks. A few years ago, I committed to breaking this habit because multitasking exacerbates my symptoms. First, I had to work on becoming mindful of what I was doing because unless I consciously paid attention, I was almost always unaware that I was doing more than one thing at a time. I'd be surfing the web while talking on the phone or editing some writing while trying to follow a movie on TV or composing an email while listening to an audiobook *and* eating a snack!

I've been surprised at how much time and discipline it's taking for me to change. My goal is to limit myself to one activity at a time. I've even felt mild anxiety arise at times when I do this; I take it as a sign of just how deeply ingrained this multitasking habit is. But in those moments when I'm only doing *one thing*, I've noticed that being fully engaged in the activity allows me to enjoy and savor it, much more than if it were competing for attention with two or three other things.

Experiment with performing tasks in slow motion.

I recommend trying this with a variety of activities: getting dressed, brushing your teeth, cooking a meal, doing the dishes, surfing the internet. Slow yourself down by about 25 percent. As with cutting back on multitasking, you may find this difficult to do. When I try it, if I'm not vigilant, I slowly start moving faster and faster until I'm back to my normal speed.

Moving in slow motion doesn't just help with symptom relief. I've also discovered that several tasks I hadn't liked before became both interesting and enjoyable. How many times have you washed the dishes without paying any attention to what you're doing? The answer for me: countless. Slowing the task down by 25 percent grounds me in the present moment so that I can enjoy the physical sensation of the warm suds on my hands and the sight of shiny clean plates and silverware as I rinse them off.

Stimulate your parasympathetic nervous system.

Two branches of the autonomic nervous system—which regulates many bodily systems without our conscious direction—are the sympathetic nervous system and the parasympathetic nervous system.

When the sympathetic nervous system is aroused, it puts you on high alert, often called the "fight-or-flight" response. The sympathetic nervous system is necessary to your survival because it enables you to respond quickly when there's a threat. In contrast, when the parasympathetic nervous system is aroused, it produces a feeling of relaxation and calm in the mind and the body.

The two systems work together; as one becomes more active, the other becomes less active. But they can get out of balance. Many people live in a constant state of high alert—or sympathetic nervous system arousal—even though there's no immediate threat.

Three recognized causes for this are our fast-paced, never-enough-time-to-do-everything lifestyle; sensory overload (exacerbated by multitasking); and the media's distorted but relentless suggestion that danger lurks around every corner.

When the sympathetic nervous system is in a state of constant arousal, the parasympathetic nervous system—the one that produces a calm and relaxed state—is underactive. By stimulating the parasympathetic nervous system, you can restore the balance and, with that balance restored, you naturally slow down your pace of life.

The following techniques for stimulating the parasympathetic nervous system are adapted from Rick Hanson's excellent book *Buddha's Brain.* You can try these just about anywhere, anytime.

- Breathe from your diaphragm. This stimulates the parasympathetic nervous system because it slows down your breathing. If you put your hand on your stomach and it rises up and down slightly as you breathe, you know you're diaphragm breathing. (This is why it's sometimes called abdominal breathing.)
- Combine diaphragm breathing with mindfulness. Gently rest your attention on whatever is happening in the present moment. If your sympathetic nervous system is in a constant state of arousal, mindfulness helps restore the proper balance between the sympathetic and parasympathetic systems by increasing the activity of the latter. This creates a feeling of calm and relaxation.
- Use imagery to stimulate the parasympathetic nervous system. Visualize yourself in a peaceful place, such as a mountain stream, a forest, or a secluded beach. Engage all your senses in this imagery—sights, sounds, the feel of the breeze on your face.

▸ Lightly run one or two fingers over your lips. Parasympathetic fibers are spread throughout your lips, so touching them stimulates the parasympathetic nervous system. I was skeptical of this until I tried it. Now it's my go-to practice for immediately calming my mind and body. Once I'm calm, I slow down naturally.

Mindfulness and slowing down are wonderfully reciprocal because each one facilitates the arising of the other. Being mindfully aware of our present-moment experience makes it easier to remember to slow down. And the more we slow down, the more mindfully aware we become of what life is offering us at the moment. Even if that offering is not exactly what we wish it would be, we can work on savoring it anyway as part of the full range of life's experiences.

33

Appreciating the Wondrousness
of the Human Body

*To be alive in this beautiful, self-organizing universe—
to participate in the dance of life with senses to perceive it,
lungs that breathe it, organs that draw nourishment
from it—is a wonder beyond words.*

—JOANNA MACY

IT WASN'T UNTIL I became chronically ill that it dawned on me
that the human body is a truly remarkable organism. As an aca-
demic, I'd lived mostly in my mind, not my body. I knew that I
depended on my body for survival, but I had very little felt-sense of
it. My newfound appreciation for this extraordinary organism led
me to devise a practice that focuses on the workings of the human
body.

It's a simple mindfulness practice. I consciously bring my awareness to one of my bodily systems or organs. Then I think about
how it functions, while vividly picturing it in action. One of the
wonders of our internal bodily systems and organs is that, even

though they're vital to our survival, we rarely notice their functioning unless we intentionally focus attention on them.

My favorite subjects for this contemplation are the circulatory system and the heart, the respiratory system and the lungs, and the excretory system (yup, you read that last one correctly).

The Circulatory System and the Heart

The circulatory system is like a network of highways inside the body that allows blood to reach each of our billions of cells. Blood brings us nutrients, water, and oxygen, and (as we'll see under the excretory system) takes away waste, such as carbon monoxide.

So this is my first contemplation: I picture the blood flowing through the thousands upon thousands of miles of blood vessels in my body, bringing to every cell the substances it needs to sustain life. I like to picture its work in detail, so I imagine it bringing nutrients, water, and oxygen to the tips of my earlobes, to my lips, and out to each finger and toe.

Just as cars on the highway must be powered in order to move, our blood needs something to move it. Our hearts, of course, provide this power. To move the blood, the heart beats about 100,000 times a day. It's about the size of a fist and yet, with a simple pumping action that we experience as a heartbeat, it keeps the blood flowing through 60,000 miles of blood vessels—yes, 60,000 miles! What an amazing organ. And so, as a second contemplation, I picture the heart as a muscle, pumping blood all around my body.

The Respiratory System

The heart is also part of the respiratory system. The heart pumps oxygen-depleted blood to the lungs where the blood picks up oxygen from the air we inhale. Then the heart pumps this oxygen-enriched blood throughout the body on the circulatory system's highway of blood vessels.

To contemplate the respiratory system in action, I picture the air from my in-breath going down to my lungs, being picked up by the heart's pumping action, and then being sent to the cells in my body. Again, I like to imagine this work in detail, so I picture the oxygen reaching every part of my body—my scalp, my chest, my abdomen, my arms and legs... everywhere.

The Excretory System

The excretory system gets rid of poisons and toxins from the body—waste that, if not removed, could do us serious harm. Although the primary organs of excretion are the lungs, kidneys, and skin, once again, the heart plays a vital role. The same pumping action of the heart that brings nutrients, water, and oxygen *to* our cells also takes harmful cellular waste *away* from our cells and delivers it to one of the organs of excretion.

If the waste is gaseous, the heart pumps it to the lungs to be excreted mostly as carbon monoxide when we exhale. If the waste is dead cells or sweat, the heart pumps it to the skin (the skin being the largest organ in the body). If it's liquid waste, the heart pumps it to the kidneys. The heart is one busy organ! As my final contemplation, I picture the circulating blood picking up waste and toxins from everywhere in my body and taking them to the proper organ for disposal, so that my body stays as poison-and-toxin-free as possible.

Those are the three bodily systems that I include in this mindfulness practice. I could easily add others to my list, such as the digestive system, the reproductive system, the nervous system. Or I could contemplate and picture these remarkable features of my body:

- The 20–23 feet of my small intestine
- The 52 bones in my two feet (that's a quarter of the bones in my body)
- The 36 muscles involved in making various facial expressions
- The 30,000–40,000 skin cells I'm shedding every hour

A final note. I'm aware that some of you have bodily systems whose functioning is impaired. I do myself. Some days my heartbeat is so prominent, it feels as if my heart is beating on the outside of my body. It's not a pleasant sensation but, then again, the function of mindfulness is to make us aware of our present-moment experience, whether it's pleasant or not.

The value of being aware of the present moment is that we're more likely to make wise choices. For example, if I'm practicing this contemplation on a day when my heartbeat is uncomfortably strong, I'll choose to emphasize the *caring* aspect of mindfulness. With care and compassion for my discomfort, I think about how, despite the discomfort, my heart is doing an extraordinary job of keeping me alive.

Mindful contemplation of the wondrousness of the human body never fails to leave me in a state of awe. I hope you'll try it.

VII. For Family, Friends, Caregivers,
and Anyone Concerned about Chronic Illness

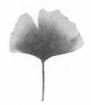

34

Setting the Record Straight about Chronic Illness

Respond intelligently even to unintelligent treatment.

—LAO TZU

IT'S IMPOSSIBLE to write honestly about life with chronic pain and illness without the subject of misconceptions coming up. The challenge of responding skillfully to the emotional pain of being misunderstood by those around us is a theme that runs throughout this book, because it's a challenge that the chronically ill face at almost every turn.

To find a measure of peace in life, we have to live as anger-free as possible, even in the midst of being misunderstood. This is not easy. With practice, however, we can learn to mindfully notice when anger has arisen; then we can consciously and intentionally choose not to feed the anger.

The Buddha said that anger directed at another comes right back to us like fine dust thrown against the wind. This is certainly true for me. That fine dust comes right back at me in the form of emotional distress and, more often than not, intensified physical symptoms.

My intention in discussing these misconceptions is twofold: to educate people about chronic illness, and to help those of us who have been misunderstood realize that we're not alone. Knowing that others who are chronically ill face the same challenges I do has greatly eased the emotional pain that can so easily accompany this unexpected turn my life has taken.

Misconception: Unless an illness is terminal, doctors can fix it.

This is what I thought before I became chronically ill. I assumed that if I got sick, all I had to do was go to the doctor, maybe get a blood test, and then I'd be given something to fix me right up. And so when I initially got sick in Paris in 2001, I went straight to a doctor. She gave me antibiotics as a precaution, even though she thought it was a viral infection. As a result, I figured I had all my bases covered: if it was viral, it would go away on its own; if it was bacterial, the antibiotics would knock it down. I assumed I'd get better and so did everyone around me. We waited... and waited... and waited... but I never recovered. Some people I know still don't understand why doctors can't fix me.

Related to this misconception is the view held by many doctors that a patient who complains of illness or pain that is not diagnosable through blood tests or other lab work has a mental disorder, such as somatization, or hypochondria. This misconception is fed by the training given to prospective doctors; they're taught to *examine, diagnose,* and (if it's not terminal) *fix.* But not all chronic illnesses can be explained by testing methods that are currently available to medical science.

Doctors should also be taught that good medical care can include saying to a patient: "I'm terribly sorry, but I don't know what's causing your symptoms; however, I'll continue to work with you to try and find an answer." Thinking back on the two dozen or so doctors I've seen since becoming chronically ill, only one has said this to me.

Misconception: If people look good, they must feel good.

It boosts most people's morale to try and look nice when they go out—whether they're chronically ill or not. I go out so seldom that I make an effort to look my best when I do. Sometimes I feel like a young child again, playing dress-up. That said, I always hope that if I see people I know, they'll remember that looks can be deceiving. Here is a portion of a comment left at the end of one of my online articles:

> I was bed bound for an extended period but have been ambulatory for the last couple of years. Those close to me and friends around me see my ability to get out of bed as a "completely healed" status. What they don't see is that I still have 24/7 pain that throbs from head to toe. I still have gastrointestinal trouble and cognition problems. I push to be part of making memories with family and friends because without that there is just suffering and tears. No one sees the dark, lonely middle of the night where I can release the tears of pain and frustration from overdoing myself.

This comment touched me deeply. I've had similar experiences when people see me outside the house. They say, "You look great." I know they're trying to be nice, so I make an effort to respond graciously—with something other than a snarky "Well I don't *feel* great." Yet the truth is, as I stand before them "looking great," my muscles are aching and my heart is pounding so hard that sometimes I'm convinced it must be visible on the outside of my body.

When people see someone who is struggling with his or her health, I hope they'll remember that they, too, have days when they leave the house looking great but feeling terrible, perhaps from a bad night's sleep or from lingering symptoms of an acute illness. And I hope this reflection will help them understand that a chronically ill person can look fine but feel awful.

Misconception: A given chronic illness manifests the same way in every person.

People can have the same diagnosis but suffer from different symptoms. Or they can have the same symptoms but at different levels of intensity. In addition, people often respond differently to the same treatment. The misconception that any given chronic illness will present with the same symptoms or will respond similarly to the same treatments leads to misunderstandings that can be hard for the chronically ill to handle skillfully. I know; I've had dozens of people say or write to me something along these lines: "I know someone who had what you have. She took [fill in the blank] and is fine now."

It's frustrating when people presume to know more about our chronic illness than we do. And yet, as challenging as these kinds of interactions can be, we should be mindful not to feed any anger that might start to arise; we don't want it to fly back at us like fine dust thrown against the wind! Instead, we can remind ourselves that others are acting out of ignorance, and that they're almost always well-intentioned and genuinely trying to help. Then we can try to change the subject.

Misconception: People are either healthy or they're sick.

Many people with chronic illnesses—including life-threatening ones—go through periods of remission. Most people don't understand this. They assume that we're either sick or we're not. For instance, since the late 1980s, I've suffered from a painful bladder condition called interstitial cystitis, which can be in remission for months at a time. I can even talk myself into thinking that this is no longer one of my chronic conditions. So far, however, after every remission, it has returned with a vengeance, and the pain can be intense.

Some chronic illnesses are episodic. People with chronic migraines—in addition to having to endure the excruciating pain of a headache—have accompanying symptoms that include nausea, vertigo, loss of hearing, and even loss of speech. Yet when they're between episodes, they're likely to feel fine, and so people forget that they suffer from a debilitating condition.

Misconception: If people's illnesses and pain conditions were truly physically based, their mental states wouldn't affect their physical symptoms.

If you're not sick or in pain, I invite you to try this simple two-part mindfulness exercise, so you can test this misconception out for yourself.

Part I: The next time you feel under stress—maybe you're on a tight deadline or you're worried about a family member—stop, close your eyes, and turn your attention to how your body feels. You'll probably notice that your muscles have tightened and your heart is beating faster. Your entire body may be pulsating, and you may even have broken out in a sweat. These are just a few of the ways that mental stress manifests in the body of a healthy person.

Part II: Keeping that stressful mental state in the forefront of your awareness, now imagine that you suffer from chronic pain or illness. What would happen? Your body would respond to the mental stress the same way it did for you as a healthy person. But now that response would be *in addition to* your chronic, everyday symptoms. And if those symptoms happen to overlap with the physical symptoms that accompany mental stress—tightened muscles, racing heart, pulsating body, and maybe even sweating—you can see how a person's mental state can easily exacerbate the physical symptoms of chronic illness.

This is why keeping mental stress to a minimum is so important for the chronically ill. Important, but often impossible. Why? Because we live in the same stressful world that healthy people live in.

Misconception: Carefully resting for days before an event will assure that when the occasion arrives, the chronically ill will be in better shape than had they not rested.

I can rest for several days in a row before a commitment and yet, on the day of the event, feel terribly sick. Resting may increase the odds that I'll be less sick than usual on the day of the event, but it's no guarantee.

When my granddaughter Cam turned six a few years ago, I asked my husband to take me to her birthday party for a short time since it's only an hour's drive away. It would have been a treat to watch her interacting with her friends—something I never get to see—and to meet their parents. I rested for four days before the event. But that morning, in tears, I called my son Jamal to tell him that I was too sick to attend.

This misconception about the effects of intense rest can lead to serious misunderstandings. For example, a week after Cam's birthday party, I was able to attend an event that was scheduled to coincide with the release of my book *How to Wake Up*. This could make it appear that I was choosing the book event over my granddaughter's party, even though I was not (and thankfully Jamal understood this).

The bottom line: the same amount of resting before each of the two events simply did not yield the same results. The unpredictability that comes with living day in and day out with chronic illness can lead to deep disappointment and sadness with our lives. If we don't treat ourselves kindly and with compassion, this unpredictability can also lead to painful feelings of self-recrimination and guilt.

Misconception: If people who are chronically ill are laughing and having a good time, they must feel fine.

When an important occasion arises, people who are chronically ill have learned to bear the symptoms of illness, including intense pain. They do this partly to try and have a good time and partly not to interfere with other people's ability to enjoy the occasion. Please don't assume that a person who is laughing is a person who is pain-free, ache-free, or otherwise feeling good physically.

Misconception: Being home all day is a dream lifestyle.

When healthy people entertain this thought, they're not contemplating being home all day *feeling sick and in pain*! Put another way, would they say "I wish I could be home all day with pain that no medicine can relieve" or "I wish I could be home all day with such debilitating fatigue that I can't even read a good book"? I doubt it.

Many years ago, I spent a long, cold winter in Winnipeg, Manitoba, where I learned a new expression for the effects of being stuck in your home day after day: "cabin fever." That winter, this California girl was repeatedly asked, "Do you have cabin fever yet?" In fact, I did, and we moved back to California as soon as the spring thaw hit.

Chronic illness leaves me mostly housebound. On the whole, I've made my peace with it. That said, I still occasionally get cabin fever. Some people find the confinement so difficult that it leads to serious emotional problems. In fact, an alternative name for cabin fever came to my attention that winter in Winnipeg: prairie madness.

Another reason that being housebound isn't a dream lifestyle is that people assume we're spending the day at leisure. I'm not, and I know many other chronically ill people who aren't either. I'm working. Writing this book is work. Responding to the hundreds of emails I get a month from people is work. Many people who are housebound by chronic illness are taking care of other family members, from little children to elderly parents. And, of course, it's work just to stay on top of our medical conditions—keeping abreast of the latest developments, assessing doctors, evaluating the effectiveness of treatments, and keeping family and friends informed about how we're doing.

In the same way we've come to think of stay-at-home moms or dads as working people, those of us who've had to leave the outside-the-house workforce due to chronic illness are still working, even if it isn't paid work. So when people say to us about our lives, "I wish I could lie around all day and do nothing," we know they just don't get it. Being at home (and often in bed) all day is not a dream lifestyle.

I've worked hard to find a measure of peace in the midst of feeling misunderstood. On the one hand, I've learned that expecting everyone to understand what my life is like sets me up for disappointment and unhappiness. On the other hand, I'm not content to always be a passive onlooker, letting misconception after misconception go unchallenged.

And so I've tried to find a middle ground. I take action to educate people about what life is like for the chronically ill and for me personally; at the same time, I work on not being attached to the results of those actions. I keep in mind that sometimes I'll succeed and sometimes I won't. This is an equanimity practice. In the context of misconceptions and misunderstandings about chronic illness, equanimity refers to being aware that not everyone will understand what life for us is like. In fact, not everyone will even be willing to make the effort to understand.

This is the way people are and always have been. It doesn't mean we should abandon our attempts to dispel the many misconceptions about life with chronic illness, and yet, even as we do that, we can work on acknowledging without bitterness that we won't always succeed. The more we can ride our disappointments with an even-tempered acceptance, the better chance we have of finding peace of mind with our circumstances.

Groucho Marx famously said that he wouldn't want to belong to a club that would have him as a member. Well, membership in the club of the chronically ill is neither voluntary nor planned. One day I wasn't a member; the next day I was. My task is to make the best of the life I've been given, while at the same time doing what I can to turn these common misconceptions into uncommon ones.

35

What the Chronically Ill Hope
Others Will Understand

One of the most beautiful qualities of true friendship
is to understand and to be understood.

—SENECA

I KNOW WHAT I hope the people in my life will understand about
me. What has surprised me is that, of the thousands of people who've written to me about living with chronic illness, almost
every one of them has the very same wishes.

This chapter is written out of love for my family and friends, and
with deep appreciation for everyone who cares about those who
suffer from chronic illness.

**We can feel as if we're letting you down even though you've
repeatedly assured us that we're not.**

I could fill a notebook with examples from my own life, but I'll
restrict myself to one. I have a weekly commitment so see my
friend Richard for a short visit at a local café. I go there instead

of inviting him over because I think it's good for me to get out of the house. He's assured me many times that any day I'm too sick, I should cancel—even at the last minute—and he won't feel let down. I believe him. He's the type of person who wouldn't say it if he didn't mean it. Despite this, I always feel as if I'm failing him or disappointing him when I cancel. This is completely irrational on my part; even so, it's how I feel.

A few months ago, I woke up one day and knew immediately that I'd have to cancel our visit. I dashed off an email to him, and we rescheduled for the next day. But the next day, I was no better. He would have wanted me to cancel again, but I didn't. Instead, I dragged myself to our usual meeting place because I couldn't shake the feeling that I'd be letting him down if I cancelled again, even though, as I've said, I believe him when he says that I would not be.

On my way home from our visit, I realized that I was holding myself to a higher standard than I'd impose on any of my friends who were chronically ill. If I had a date with a friend who was sick or in pain, I'd feel the same way Richard feels about me—I'd want that friend to cancel. And yet I had insisted on pushing myself beyond what my body could handle. It would have been an act of self-compassion to have cancelled that day. I'm aware of that now, and I'm trying to change.

We may apologize for being sick and for being in pain even though you don't want us to.

I'm surprised that after so many years of being sick, I can still find myself apologizing to people for not being able to do things and for the ways my illness has affected our relationship. I apologize even though they're not expecting me to and even though they don't want me to. Again, this is irrational, but I still do it.

In 2013, our friend Nhi drove two hours from San Francisco to go out to lunch with my husband and me. When she arrived, I was too sick to go. I told her that she and my husband would have to go to lunch on their own and that I'd visit with her for a bit when they returned. I told her this—but not before profusely apologizing for not being able to go to lunch.

Nhi knew when we made the plans that I might not be able to go, but she was willing to take the risk anyway. She used to be our neighbor, so she's seen me at my worst. In fact, she's *only* known me as a person who struggles every day with chronic illness. She didn't expect or want an apology, but I issued one anyway.

When my son Jamal and his family come to spend the day with us, there's no need for me to apologize when I have to retire to the bedroom. But I do anyway. My husband is so used to my unnecessary apologies that he can look at my face and sense that one is on the way. More than once, before I've been able to get the words "I'm sorry I got sick" out of my mouth, he's already saying, "You don't need to apologize. It's not your fault that you're sick."

I've decided that it makes me feel better to apologize. It's my way of saying, "I know that the effect of this illness on our relationship and on my inability to participate fully in whatever you're doing is no fun for you either." So to those who care about us: please forgive us for apologizing so much (there I go, apologizing for apologizing!).

Talking about our health can be uncomfortable for us.

The state of my health feels like it should be a private matter, even from those I feel close to. Most people keep the intimate details of their lives private. Why not chronic illness? The answer is that most of us don't have the luxury of keeping our medical conditions private. We have to explain to people why we can't do this and why we can't do that; why we have to cancel plans at the last minute; why we have to suddenly sit down or leave a gathering early.

And so, instead of keeping this intimate part of our lives private, we're forced to talk about it.

In addition, some chronic illnesses have symptoms that are embarrassing to talk about, such as Crohn's disease or irritable bowel syndrome. As I mentioned in the previous chapter, I suffer from a painful bladder condition called interstitial cystitis. I try to keep it private, even from those I'm closest to. I'm not comfortable talking about how the walls of my bladder can feel as if they're allergic to urine. And yet sometimes I have to share that I have this condition so I can explain some of my peculiar behavior, such as why my first priority upon entering a building is to figure out where the nearest restroom is.

Finally, the economic consequences of chronic illness feel as if they should be private. I know many chronically ill people who have been forced to move back in with a parent because they're no longer able to care for themselves, or because they can no longer afford to live independently. Sometimes a parent must move in with a child for the same reasons. These matters feel as if they should be kept between family members, but that's often not possible. If nothing else, friends need to know where we're living! Sharing the economic consequences of being chronically ill can be so uncomfortable for us that it can give rise to feelings of shame.

We may at times be irrational about our health... and our lives.

Some days, the intensity of my physical symptoms makes it hard for me to think clearly. I can get so discouraged that I blow things way out of proportion. For example, if my symptoms flare one day, instead of waiting until morning to see if I feel a bit better, I'll panic and announce to my husband in no uncertain terms that this is my new normal. Or if a friend cancels a visit, I'll jump to the conclusion that she no longer wants to hang out with someone who's sick all the time.

Sometimes this irrational behavior takes the form of discounting the positives in order to focus on the negatives. If my son Jamal and his family are visiting on a day when I'm particularly sick, I might dwell on how bad I feel about the things we can no longer do together, instead of paying attention to what we *can* do. Discounting the positives in this way detracts from the good time we could be having in each other's company.

I can even do more than discount the positives. I can turn them into negatives! I'm not the only chronically ill person who does this; it appears that the worse we feel physically, the more likely we are to engage in this irrational behavior. For example, I might get an email from a friend who hasn't written to me in a long time. Instead of feeling good about her gesture, I'll turn it into a negative experience: "She only emailed me out of obligation, not because she really wants to stay in touch." It's my husband who usually has to listen to me transform into a negative experience the simple fact that someone was kind enough to send me an email.

We know how hard this irrational and distorted thinking is on those who care about us and, yup, we apologize.

We're grateful that you accept our chronic illness and have adjusted to it; even so, we hope you won't forget that we can still suffer terribly, both physically and mentally.

Several people have shared with me that a friend or relative has started to treat their chronic illness as routine and, as a result, has become desensitized to it. I've had this happen, and I've decided that it's understandable. When those who care deeply about us must continually witness the effects of our illness on every part of our lives together, we can't expect them to always be at their empathetic best. Nevertheless, this doesn't lessen our concern that the people on whom we count for emotional support will become so accustomed to our being sick and to our being in pain that they'll forget that our physical suffering and our sorrow can be as intense now as it was when we first became chronically ill.

In June of 2014, my son's and daughter's families met up at Disneyland so that my two granddaughters, Cam and Malia, could spend the day together at the Park. Given where the two families live, it's rare for all of them to be together like this—so rare that my husband drove from Northern California to Southern California so he could be part of this special day. Thankfully, many people who are chronically ill are still able to travel. Unfortunately, I am not, and so I stayed home.

I wanted my family to have a wonderful time at Disneyland. Even so, I couldn't help but hope that they understood how painful it was for me to miss this special occasion. I'm not alone in this wish. We who are chronically ill hope that the people in our lives won't come to view our medical condition as such a normal state of affairs that they'll forget to give us that extra hug or once in a while say to us, "I'm so sorry this has happened."

The grief we feel over the life we've lost may reemerge indefinitely.

I've read several studies that list the most stressful events in people's lives. Regardless of who conducted the study, certain events appear on every list. Serious illness is one of them. It's considered a grief-producing event, just as are other major life losses, such as the loss of a relationship due to separation or death.

Until I became chronically ill, I had no idea that the people I knew who had ongoing health struggles were grieving. Now I know that there's a lot to mourn—the loss of the capacity to be as productive as we once were, the loss of friends, the loss of the ability to take part in cherished activities, the loss of independence.

We hope that the people we know will understand that grief comes in waves. It can arrive unexpectedly, throwing us off guard.

One moment, we can feel accepting of the changes in our lives. The next moment we can be overcome by sadness.

In addition, grief can be triggered by a seemingly innocuous interaction. For example, I thought I was done mourning over my lost career. It's been over a decade since I had to stop working due to illness. Then, one day, a former colleague came into the café where I was waiting to meet my friend Dawn. She sat down and began to describe all the changes that have taken place at the law school where I taught. To my surprise, a wave of grief overcame me, and I had to try hard not to break out in tears in front of her. This was particularly unexpected since, were I to recover, I wouldn't return to my old profession.

The words of Sameet Kumar in his book *Grieving Mindfully* have been comforting to me when unexpected grieving confuses and even confounds me:

> Grief is the process of finding out who you are in a world that is barely recognizable because of the tremendous change that has taken place.

The grieving process I've gone through as a result of chronic illness has been intense at times. Odd as it may sound, it's been more intense than the grief I felt when my mother died. She lived across the Atlantic from me, and we rarely saw each other. She had a long, good life. I was sad to lose her, and, yes, I grieved, yet it was not the lengthy and deep grieving I've gone through over the upheaval in my life due to chronic illness.

We want to be treated as your equals on the path of life.

The American mythologist Joseph Campbell said:

The big question is whether you are going to be able to say a hearty yes to your adventure.

Whether chronically ill or not, all of us face the challenge posed by his words. Everyone's life is a series of unique adventures with ups and downs, successes and disappointments, joys and sorrows. I want the people in my life to share with me what's going on with them—tough times included—so we can help each other say a *hearty yes*, and so we can say it together, as equals on the path of life.

36

"Oh No!": What the Chronically Ill Hope Others Won't Say

*One's dignity may be assaulted, vandalized, and cruelly mocked,
but it can never be taken away unless it is surrendered.*

—MICHAEL J. FOX

THE PURPOSE of this chapter is not to make those whose comments are off the mark feel bad. Even the most well-intentioned people often don't know how to talk to the chronically ill. This is because we live in a culture that treats illness as unnatural. As a result, people have been conditioned to turn away in aversion from those who aren't healthy, even though it's a fate that will befall everyone at some point in his or her life.

The consequences of taking this unrealistic view of the realities of the human condition is that many people feel uneasy and even fearful when they encounter people who are struggling with their health. I admit that this was true of me before I became chronically ill. Now I find it as natural to talk to people who are chronically ill as I do to people who are the pinnacle of health.

I hope this chapter encourages people who know someone who is chronically ill to become more mindful of their speech. I also hope it will help those who are sick and those who are in pain feel less alone. I expect that those of you who are chronically ill will recognize many of the comments you're about to read.

The first twelve comments have been made to me at least once since I became ill in 2001. They are followed by a collection of comments that other people have sent to me, comments that they said were, at best, not helpful and, at worst, extremely hurtful.

"You look fantastic!"

It's a challenge to respond to comments such as "You look fantastic" or the dreaded "But you don't *look* sick," because we know that the speaker is only trying to be nice. If we respond truthfully with "Well, I don't *feel* fantastic" or "Thanks, but I feel awful," the other person might be embarrassed or think we're being ungrateful. I admit that I've never come up with a satisfactory response to this comment. I usually mumble "thanks" and try to change the subject.

"You just need to get out more often."

One day, my husband and I were at an espresso place and a woman who knows I'm sick stopped and said to me, "You look so good!" My husband politely responded that actually, I was quite sick. When she then said to me, "You just need to get out more often," I was at a loss for words. My husband told me afterward that he wanted to say to her, "You don't heal a broken leg by going for a hike." He held his tongue because he thought she might take it as an insult.

"Give me a call if there's anything I can do."

I've been on the receiving end of this well-intentioned comment many times. Not once has it resulted in my picking up the phone.

The offer is too open-ended. It puts the ball in my court and I'm not going to hit it back, either because I'm too proud, too shy, too sick—or a combination of the three. I'm not going to call and say, "Can you come over and weed my garden?" But if someone were to call and offer to come over and do it, I'll gratefully say, "Yes!"

"I wish I could lie around all day and do nothing."

I mentioned this comment in chapter 34. A friend said it to me over the phone; it's stuck in my mind all these years because it hurt terribly at the time. It may sound as if it couldn't possibly have been well-intentioned and yet, given the tone of voice in which it was delivered, I've decided it was. I'm sure that my high-powered, overworked friend was genuinely thinking, "Lucky you to have so much leisure time."

When she said it, I was still so sensitive about being sick—including being worried that people might think I was a malingerer—that tears came to my eyes. I wanted to scream at her, "You have no idea how it feels to be stuck in bed and have no choice *but* to do nothing!" Instead, I mumbled something and made an excuse to get off the phone because I could feel the sobs coming—which they did as soon as I hung up.

"Disease is a message from your soul, telling you that something is wrong with your True Self."

This is an excerpt from one of dozens of emails I've received from people trying to diagnose or cure me. I must admit that I have no idea what the sentence means. Are the soul and the True Self different entities, and the one that is okay is sending a message to the other one saying that something's wrong with it? Bottom line: This is not helpful. And while we're on the subject of "not helpful," another person said she'd help me get my health back—free of charge—by showing me how to perform a "soul retrieval." Sigh.

"My sister-in-law's best friend had what you have and said she got better by drinking bottled water."

Little did this speaker realize that it's just as likely that my own sister-in-law's best friend had what I have and told me that I could get better if I *stopped* drinking bottled water! It would be such a relief if people understood that, despite their best intentions, we're unlikely to want advice on treatments—unless we ask for it, of course. Most of us have spent hours on the internet, researching possible treatments. We know what's available, and we know what we're considering. When people offer treatments, especially based on anecdotal evidence, it puts us in a position of having to defend our treatment decisions.

Another piece of treatment advice that many of us have heard multiple times: "Have you tried sleeping pills?" Sleeping pills? Who hasn't tried sleeping pills? Even healthy people do. Sleeping pills may be helpful for some people, but they are not a cure for chronic illness. Regarding any comment that starts with the phrase "Have you tried… ": If it's available by prescription or as a supplement or even as a Chinese herb, the odds are very high that I know about it and that I've tried it!

"Do you meditate?"

Yes, I meditate—although, depending on our relationship, this may be an intrusive question. Meditation and other stress-reduction techniques (some of which you'll find in this book) can help with symptom relief and with the mental stress that often accompanies ongoing pain and illness. However, they are not a cure for a physically based chronic illness.

"Aren't you worried that you're getting out of shape from living such a sedentary lifestyle?"

Uh… yes. Thanks for reminding me.

"Just don't think about it."

This comment left me speechless... but still thinking about "it."

"Are you eating enough fruits and vegetables?"

As many as this one body can hold!

"Have you Googled your symptoms?"

Let me count the ways.

"At least you still have your sense of humor."

Thanks. Truth be told, however, I'd rather be a humorless healthy person.

Here are comments that others have written to me about. Many of them were passed on to me by multiple people. I've divided them into five categories: *Change Your Lifestyle, Such an Easy Life, Chronic Means Chronic, It's Your Fault,* and *Religion and other Spiritual Matters.*

Change Your Lifestyle

1. *"Do you take vitamins?"* Who hasn't tried vitamins?

2. *"Just eat more."*

3. *"Just eat less."*

4. *"Are you drinking water?"*

5. *"All you need is some fresh air and exercise."*

6. *"Why don't you go to bed earlier?"*

7. *"Why don't you take a shower? You'll feel better."* This one hit

home for me because I have days when taking a shower has the opposite effect: this simple task uses up all my energy stores for the day.

Such an Easy Life

1. *"You have such an easy life!"* Several people have told me how hurtful this comment is—and how hard it is to respond to without getting angry.

2. *"You're lucky to have so much leisure time!"* Wrote another woman: "Yeah, it's great to have so much time, but I'm unable to work. This puts me so far below the poverty line that homeless people begging for change probably have more money at their disposal than I do." Many people who are chronically ill are living below the poverty line. A combination of causes is at work here. They may have been abandoned by their partners; they may no longer be able to hold down a job. Or both. In addition, the chronically ill often have to spend what money they *do* have on medications and other treatments that health insurance doesn't cover. Tragically, poverty and chronic illness too often go hand-in-hand.

3. *"I wish I didn't have to work!"* One woman wrote, "It's like telling someone without legs they're lucky they don't have to take the stairs."

Chronic Means Chronic

1. *"You're STILL in pain?"* or *"You're STILL sick?"* Yes, we're still in pain and we're still sick—chronic means chronic!

2. *"Don't worry, you'll be able to go hiking again soon."* I've had people make similar remarks to me about various activities—from traveling to resuming my teaching career. If you're not sure what

your friend might or might not be able to do in the future, it's better not to raise it.

3. *"Call me when you feel better, and we'll go to lunch or do something fun."* Again, chronic means chronic.

4. *"My mother-in-law had that and all she did was take a little Tylenol."* Ah, yes. Tylenol—that well-known cure for chronic illness.

It's Your Fault

1. *"You're too young to be sick."* So many people reported being told this that I've devoted a chapter in this book to the difficulties faced by young people who are chronically ill. A young woman went on to tell me: "Oh, how wish I were too young. Maybe by the time I'm in my eighties, people will stop saying it."

2. *"Get a job, mingle with people, and engage your brain."* A young woman wrote to me, saying: "I'm sensitive about being perceived as lazy. I'm hurt whenever this comment is made to me. I'd love to be able to will myself to do whatever I'd like." This resonated strongly with me because I spent years trying to will my body back into good health. All I got for my effort was a dose of mental suffering on top of my physical suffering.

3. *"You must be out of alignment with your life and looking for an excuse to make some changes."* The person who reported having had to listen to this comment said, "But some of us really loved our lives before we got ill." To that, I say, "Absolutely!" I was never happier—personally and professionally—than when I got sick in 2001.

4. *"Maybe if you quit talking about it, you'll get better."*

5. *"It's all about your attitude."*

6. "*Just snap out of it.*" The woman who reported this comment went on to say: "Like it's really that simple, and I'm so totally dumb and stupid that I can't figure it out. How silly of me after so many years."

7. "*If you think of yourself as a cripple, you will become a cripple.*" This most egregious comment was made by a doctor.

Religion and Other Spiritual Matters

This is a sensitive subject. We each have our particular religious and spiritual beliefs. Understandably, they may feel essential to our well-being. In my opinion, these matters are so personal that unless you know that the person you're talking to shares your beliefs, it's better not to raise the subject. As one person told me: "The assumption that all of us have or even should have identical spiritual beliefs is unrealistic in our pluralistic society. If you're not sure you're on the same track, it might best be avoided."

Here are some comments that have been directed at those who are struggling with their health.

1. "*God never gives you more than you can handle.*" According to those who've been on the receiving end of this comment, it's worse than nonconsoling; it makes them feel like failures—as if they're not handling well what God thinks they *should* be handling well.

2. "*God is trying to teach you something.*"

3. "*If you pray to God harder and longer, He will cure you.*"

4. "*All things work for the Good for those who love God.*" The woman who reported this comment to me said this about it: "There's nothing more annoying than some random Bible quote thrown into your face as a 'reason' for chronic pain."

Comments about religion, regardless of the speaker's intent, tend to make people feel as if they're chronically ill because they're doing something wrong. For this reason, these comments also belong under the previous heading: It's Your Fault.

I recognize that this chapter contains a lot of "Don't say this" and "Don't say that" admonitions. My purpose in writing it is to help people understand what kinds of comments are difficult for the chronically ill to field tactfully and skillfully.

I've learned not to expect people to say the perfect thing. In fact, I give them a lot of leeway because, as I indicated at the beginning of this chapter, until I became chronically ill myself, I didn't know what to say to those who were sick and to those who were in pain. And so if someone's comment is off the mark, instead of saying something rude in return, I ask myself: "Did they intend to be thoughtful?" "Did they intend to make me feel better?" If the answer is yes, then I try not to take the comment personally, and I respond as graciously as I can.

If you're wondering, "So what *can* I say?" have a look at the next chapter. In addition, the Buddha offered some valuable guidance on skillful speech. He said that before you speak, reflect on whether what you're about to say is true, kind, and helpful. It's often easy to meet two of the criteria, but not all three. If you're in doubt as to whether what you're about to say is true, kind, *and* helpful, it's best to simply not make the comment. Silence (and a gentle hug) can be golden.

37

"Thank You!": What the Chronically Ill Hope Others Will Say

The most I can do for my friend is simply be his friend.

—HENRY DAVID THOREAU

A s a follow-up to the previous chapter, I thought it would be helpful to consider what the chronically ill wish others *would* say to them. What follows are comments that would be music to my ears. Based on what people who are chronically ill have told me, I'm not alone in hoping to hear these words.

"You look good, but how are you really feeling?"

Compare this to the first example in the previous chapter: "You look fantastic!" Not only does the word "good" sound more authentic than the overblown "fantastic," but it would be such a relief to be asked a question that goes to the heart of the matter: "How are you *really* feeling?"

"I'm going to the grocery store; can I pick anything up for you?"

This is helpful, as opposed to the more common "Call me if there's anything I can do" mentioned in the previous chapter. As I said there, we're unlikely to take you up on such an open-ended offer; that is, we're not going to call and ask, "Can you go to the grocery store and get me some dish soap?" We don't want to make people go somewhere they aren't otherwise going. On the other hand, if they let us know that they're *already* going to the store, that's a different matter entirely!

In fact, the more specific an offer of help is, the better. For example, we'd love to hear an offer to do one of those life tasks that backs up for us because we're not well enough to get to it: take our car for an oil change (we'll pay for it), rake our leaves, do a load of laundry, even clean the refrigerator.

"It must be hard to be in pain so much of the time," or "Not being able to work must be so frustrating," or "I imagine it's a daily grind to have to pace yourself so carefully."

These comments are examples of "active listening," a technique I discussed in chapter 18. When you actively listening to someone, you think about how you'd feel if you were in his or her shoes. Then, using your own words, you do your best to feed those feelings back to that person.

Speaking personally, I appreciate any attempt by another person to see my life from my point of view. For example, every December, my husband, my son, and my daughter-in-law go to a holiday party given by our friends Nhi and Greg in San Francisco. It's a very festive occasion. I used to feel disappointed and terribly sad that I couldn't go but, over the years, I've made my peace with staying home. Even so, were someone to say to me, "It must be disappointing that you can't go to the holiday party with your family," I'd be grateful for his or her effort to understand what life is like for me.

It's okay if a person's words aren't right on the mark. It's the intention that matters. All of us—chronically ill or not—want to know that others are trying to understand our lives. I hope that everyone has experienced the sweet relief that comes from feeling heard and validated.

"How are you holding up? Do we need to stop visiting so you can rest?"

It would be a blessing to hear someone offer this "prompt." I've lost count of the number of times my body was telling me to lie down, but I didn't excuse myself. Even if we're wilting from fatigue or are in bad pain, many of us will try to conceal it because we don't want to let others down. But an inquiry like the one above lets us know that the person is aware of and sensitive to our limitations. That makes us feel comfortable enough to respond honestly.

"I miss going out to lunch together," or "I miss going to the movies with you," or "I miss going to the mall together."

I definitely want to hear a heartfelt expression of how my family and friends feel impacted by this drastic change in our lives together. It lets me know that they value our relationship.

"Don't feel bad if you have to cancel our plans at the last minute. I'll understand."

What a relief this would be to hear. I still sometimes force myself to keep commitments even though I'm too sick to do so. Invariably, it leads to a flare-up of symptoms, known in the chronic illness community as a "crash." I'm better than I used to be about cancelling plans if I'm having a particularly rough day. When I do cancel, I feel less bad about it if those plans were made with one of my "it's okay to cancel" friends. I treasure them.

"Would you like to hear about this crazy adventure I had yesterday?"

Indeed I would! Some people don't want to tell me about what they're up to, especially if it's something exciting. They think that talking about their lives will make me feel bad since I'm so limited in what I can do. Perhaps not everyone who is chronically ill would welcome this type of comment. For me, however, hearing about a friend's adventure makes me feel connected to the world and adds real-life experiences to what I mostly have to get off the television.

"I hope you're as well as possible."

This comment is so spot-on to those of us living day-to-day with chronic illness that we just use the initials AWAP when communicating with each other, as in, "I hope you're AWAP." Reflecting on this, wouldn't it be a compassionate comment to make to anyone? Everybody has his or her share of stresses and sorrows—in sickness *and* in health. And so my wish for all of you is that you be AWAP.

I hope that if you have a friend or family member who is chronically ill, you'll take your cue from these suggested comments when speaking to them. And please don't judge yourself negatively if you feel uncomfortable around those who are sick and those who are in pain. In this culture, most of us have never learned to treat illness as a natural and normal part of the life cycle. I hope that, instead of blaming yourself, you'll cultivate compassion for yourself over any unease or fear you're experiencing. With compassion for your discomfort as your companion, set the intention to speak in a kind and helpful way. Then muster all the courage you can and dive on in.

When I'm not sure what to say to someone who is chronically ill, I start with "I'm sorry"—because I truly *am* sorry. "I'm sorry that you're in pain" or "I'm sorry that you've been so sick lately." This is not an "I pity you" sorry. It's a compassionate sorry. Compassion means "to suffer with." And so speak in such a way that those you care about feel as if you're in this together.

38

What's in a Name? The Harm Caused by Mislabeling Medical Conditions

It's better to understand a little than to misunderstand a lot.

—ANATOLE FRANCE

L ABELS MATTER. We quickly form judgments based on them. If we hear someone described as lazy, the label "lazy person" attaches in our minds even though we may not even have met the person. The same is true for labels given to medical conditions. For example, if the label for an illness includes the word "fatigue," we abstract from our personal experience and assume we understand how a person with that illness feels.

Some medical conditions have been named after the researcher who discovered or described them in the medical literature (Alzheimer's and Crohn's). Others are named after a famous patient (Lou Gehrig's disease). The result: instant legitimacy.

The trend, however, is to name disorders by describing their signs or symptoms. Although this may make sense in some contexts, it can also lead to inaccurate labeling—which, in turn, can lead to harmful consequences. If an illness or pain condition has a trivial-sounding name, people may have their medical problems disregarded by others, including the medical establishment. In addition to the damaging emotional effect of being stigmatized in this way, the trivialization of a medical condition affects the crucial issue of how much research money will be allocated for finding effective treatments and for figuring out the causes of chronic illnesses that remain little understood.

Rheumatoid Arthritis

Rheumatoid arthritis is a good example of a medical condition in which a misleading name can lead to negative consequences for its sufferers. People with rheumatoid arthritis are often erroneously lumped together with those who have osteoarthritis. As soon as people hear the term "arthritis" they automatically think of joints that have become painful and stiff due to aging. But those symptoms describe osteoarthritis, a nagging but, for the most part, benign condition that affects almost everyone to some extent as he or she gets old. By contrast, rheumatoid arthritis is a serious systemic autoimmune disease that can occur at any age. Joint pain and stiffness are but two of its many symptoms.

The consequences of these two conditions having such similar names is that people with rheumatoid arthritis are likely to be treated as if they have osteoarthritis. This label-confusion is especially hard on young people with rheumatoid arthritis. Several young women have told me that they repeatedly have to listen to hurtful comments, such as "You're too young to have bad joint pain" or "People your age don't get arthritis."

While not considered a fatal illness, rheumatoid arthritis can shorten people's life expectancy, partly because they are at higher risk for complications such as anemia, lung disease, coronary artery disease, and lymphoma. Chemotherapy drugs (with their accompanying side-effects) are often prescribed to suppress the autoimmune reaction in people with rheumatoid arthritis.

The rheumatoid arthritis community would like to see the name changed to rheumatoid autoimmune disease. This designation would eliminate the confusion that results from being diagnosed with an illness that has the word "arthritis" in it.

Chronic Fatigue Syndrome

Although my cluster of symptoms doesn't neatly fit the various case definitions for chronic fatigue syndrome (CFS), of the diagnostic codes available to doctors, CFS comes closest to describing my illness, so "chronic fatigue syndrome" is what they put down on forms. The consensus among the specialists I've seen is that the viral infection I contracted in 2001 compromised my immune system in some way, and it no longer functions normally. However, there's no diagnostic code for immune system dysfunction, so chronic fatigue syndrome has become my official diagnosis.

The principal misleading word here is "fatigue." Every CFS sufferer I know has had to listen to others say, "I'm tired too." When they hear those words, they know that their illness has been mislabeled; even worse, they know that the stigmatizing label "malingerer" may not be far behind.

The "fatigue" of chronic fatigue syndrome bears no resemblance to the fatigue that people experience after a bad night's sleep. As many people have pointed out, calling this illness "chronic fatigue syndrome" is like calling emphysema "chronic cough syndrome" or Alzheimer's "chronic forgetfulness syndrome." The fatigue of chronic fatigue syndrome is often described as a bone-crushing fatigue. I call it bone-crushing and sickly fatigue. Laura Hillenbrand, bestselling author of *Seabiscuit* and *Unbroken* and a CFS sufferer herself, put it this way: "This illness is to fatigue what a nuclear bomb is to a match. It's an absurd mischaracterization."

I feel certain that, were it not for this woefully misleading label, the American Academy of Family Physicians (AAFP) would not have begun its recently released "Patient Information Sheet on Chronic Fatigue Syndrome" with this sentence:

> Chronic fatigue syndrome is a disorder that causes you to be very tired.

I am not "very tired." I'm not even "tired." I don't nod off while people are talking to me. I don't even fall asleep while reading or watching TV. This is because I'm not tired. I'm sick. Among other symptoms, I have the kind of sickly fatigue and malaise that healthy people suffer from when they have an acute illness like the flu—only I've felt this way since 2001. I call it "the flu without the fever."

As of this writing, there's no known cause or cure for chronic fatigue syndrome. This is not surprising, given that so little money is allocated for research into this debilitating illness. Why is this the case? One reason is the presence of the word "fatigue" in its name. It's because of that word that an association like the AAFP can say that people with CFS are "very tired." How can we expect chronic fatigue syndrome to be taken seriously as an illness when its sufferers are described as "very tired"?

On October 15, 2009, one of the foremost experts on CFS, Dr. Nancy Klimas, spoke to the *New York Times* about the lack of research money:

> My HIV patients for the most part are hale and hearty thanks to three decades of intense and excellent research and billions of dollars invested. Many of my CFS patients, on the other hand, are terribly ill and unable to work or

participate in the care of their families. I split my clinical time between the two illnesses, and I can tell you, if I had to choose between the two illnesses in 2009, I would rather have HIV.

When doctors ask what's wrong with me, I can give one of two answers, neither of which is satisfactory in the context of obtaining quality health care for myself or others with a CFS diagnosis. This leaves me in a no-win position in the doctor's office.

Option 1: If I say, "I've been diagnosed with chronic fatigue syndrome," I'm likely to be discredited as a witness to my own illness. I've had doctors tell me there's no such thing as CFS. One doctor said, "Just drink some coffee."

Option 2: If I say, "I contracted a serious viral infection and never recovered," it goes down better with the doctor, but by saying this I'm undermining the effort to bring legitimacy to the illness. And legitimacy brings with it research funding.

A few years ago, I had an appointment with a doctor regarding something unrelated to my illness. The new-patient form asked, "Are you in good health?" I checked "no." Next question: "If you checked 'no,' please explain." How many times have I faced "please explain" on a medical form and had to choose between those two unsatisfactory options? I've lost count. I needed the best care I could get from this doctor so, playing it safe, I reluctantly took option 2 and wrote, "Contracted a serious viral infection in 2001 and never recovered."

In the examining room, the doctor looked at my form and asked: "What's this viral infection you never recovered from?" Without using the phrase "chronic fatigue syndrome," I succinctly explained how a seemingly acute viral infection had turned into a chronic illness, leaving me feeling as if I had the flu all the time.

He listened and then asked, "What's the diagnosis?" I was

cornered. I replied, "chronic fatigue syndrome." I watched as he disengaged from me. He swiveled on his stool and put down his note pad. Then he turned back to me and, addressing me as if we'd just met, said, "What have you come to see me about today?"

I take back what I said in response to the AAFP characterizing me as "very tired." I *am* very tired. I'm very tired of the lack of serious attention given to this devastating illness, due in large part to its ridiculous name.

Restless Leg Syndrome

I was diagnosed with this life-disrupting neurological disorder in the early 1990s, but I rarely tell anyone. I never even told my two children. Why? Because the name is embarrassing. Let's see how accurately the label describes the condition.

Restless

When I get an attack of restless leg syndrome (RLS), my legs aren't restless. They are seized by waves of gnawing unpleasant sensations that are so unbearable I'm forced to move my legs to try and get relief. After each wave, the sensations subside, only to return in another thirty to sixty seconds. This can go on for hours. When an attack comes at night (which is when RLS most often occurs), it's impossible to sleep. The result can be a sleepless night and one very long and unpleasant day ahead.

Leg

Sometimes I get these waves of gnawing sensations in my hands. Others get them in their arms. There's nothing exclusively "leg" about restless leg syndrome.

The Federal Drug Administration has approved two prescription medications for restless leg syndrome—Requip and Mirapex. You'd think that FDA approval of two medications for a disorder would make it legitimate. Not so. The words "restless" and "leg" are just too silly. A few years ago, I heard a late night comedian make cruel fun of RLS, saying: "And now there's a drug for restless leg syndrome. Come off it. Your legs are restless? Get a life." Ironically, I only heard his comment because I was awake due to, yup, restless leg syndrome.

So I've come out of the closet: I have restless leg syndrome. On nights when the medication doesn't work, you'll find me pacing the floors, willing to try just about anything to keep the unbearable sensations from continuing. No matter how cold a night it is, I put ice on my feet and calves. Or I wrap my legs so tightly in ace bandages that I have to be careful not to cut off the blood circulation. These home remedies are only marginally helpful because they tend to work only if I catch an attack right when it starts, and RLS doesn't wake me up until it's "up and running," so to speak. That means I'm looking at another night of broken sleep.

The mislabeling of medical conditions causes a great deal of harm. It stigmatizes those who suffer from them and affects the amount of research funding that gets allocated for finding causes and treatments. Many people in the chronic illness community are determined to get these names changed. They are tireless in their efforts, sometimes engaging in advocacy from their beds. We are indebted to these warriors for their dedication and resolve.

39

Letting Go: A Not-To-Do List
for Caregivers

*We do not heal the past by dwelling there; we heal
the past by living fully in the present.*

—MARIANNE WILLIAMSON

A S I NOTED in chapter 2, I've changed from a *to-do* list maker to
a *not-to-do* list maker, because I feel better mentally and
physically when I pay careful and caring attention to what *not to
do*. I believe that the estimated forty-five million people in the US
alone who are caregivers for elderly relatives or for the chronically
ill would also benefit from a not-to-do list.

Do not pretend that everything is like it used to be.

If you're a caregiver, you may be tempted to pretend that everything is like it used to be. But it isn't. Denying this can lead to
bitterness and resentment. It's better to face it. One day you were
relatively free to go out whenever you wanted and hang out with
whomever you wanted. The next day, you were tied to the house

and expected to understand how to take care of someone who may need help with the most intimate of life functions. This is tough and can severely impact your quality of life. Our society does a poor job of preparing people for this very real possibility. The person in your care needs time to grieve; so do you.

In addition to grieving your loss of freedom, you may be mourning the loss of the relationship you once had with the person you're caring for. Before I got sick my husband and I did almost everything together, except when we were at work. Now, for the most part, he's on his own out there in the world. It took several years for him to accept this new life and to find a measure of peace and contentment with it.

If you're a caregiver, try to recognize that pretending that everything is like it used to be is a way of turning away in aversion from your life as it is right now. This turning away is a form of denial that's likely to feed a painful longing to return to a life that's no longer possible for you. This is a recipe for unhappiness.

To find peace with your new life, begin by acknowledging with care and compassion that it's natural to grieve the loss of your old life. Allowing yourself to feel the sadness that accompanies grieving paves the way for accepting your life as it is—instead of staying stuck in that painful place of pretending that everything is like it used to be.

Do not shy away from sharing with others that you've become a caregiver.

Men are particularly reluctant to share with others that they've become caregivers. They're likely to hide it at work. They often hide it from their friends. It's a sad commentary on our culture that we still haven't found a way to make men feel comfortable sharing with others that, when they're at home, they're taking care of a partner, a sibling, a parent, or a grown child. They're doing the cooking and the cleaning; they're running all the errands; they may even be providing nursing-type assistance.

One consequence of caregivers hiding their role is that people who'd be willing to help aren't aware that help is needed. This can lead to caregiver burnout, which is one reason why caregivers have such a high incidence of clinical depression. The National Family Caregiving Association found that over 60 percent of caregivers who provide at least twenty hours of caregiving a week suffer from depression.

If you're a caregiver, I hope you'll talk to others about your life. If you're the one being cared for, encourage your caregiver to share with others the difficulties he or she is facing. No one benefits from a caregiver "going it alone." It may take only one friend to make a significant difference in a caregiver's life: one friend whom he or she can confide in and talk to about how stressful and difficult life has become; one friend whom he or she can ask for help and support. "Troubles shared are troubles halved" is one of those good clichés.

Do not think you have to make the person in your care happy.

There's a tendency for caregivers to think that one of their duties is to make the person in their care feel good, if not physically, then mentally. If you're a caregiver, this is an unrealistic assessment of your powers! It's also unlikely that your loved one expects this of you. I'm grateful when my husband is simply willing to listen to me talk about how miserable I feel—physically and, sometimes, emotionally. I don't expect him to make me happy. If you're a caregiver, don't underestimate how much it means to your loved one for you to do nothing more than bear witness to what he or she going through.

Do not expect yourself to always be up for the task at hand.

Allow yourself to have days when, even though you're doing what needs to be done for the person in your care, your heart isn't in it and you wish you were free of the obligation and the burden. In other words, don't judge yourself negatively if resentment arises now and then. Like everyone else in this life, you're going to have good days and bad days.

Do not feel guilty when you're enjoying yourself.

Be on the alert for that Super Caregiver mentality that has you thinking you're not a good caregiver unless you're never having more fun than your loved one is. I *want* my husband to have a good time. It makes me feel better about the drastic changes in his life and about the responsibilities he's had to take on. As an added bonus, knowing he's having fun can make me feel good. As I noted in chapter 28 on coping with isolation, Buddhists call this mudita—feeling joy for others who are happy. What I love about this practice is that sometimes feeling happy for my husband boomerangs; it comes back at me so that I begin to feel happy myself, as if I'm having a good time *through* him.

In 2014, my husband took our granddaughter Cam to see the Harlem Globetrotters. When I was growing up, my dad took me to see the Globetrotters whenever they came to town, so it would have been a treat for me to take Cam. But I couldn't, so my husband did.

My choice was to be envious and resentful—or to be happy for him. I chose the latter. Throughout the afternoon, I imagined the two of them in their seats—he pointing out a dribbling sleight-of-hand that Cam might have missed, both of them laughing at the Globetrotters' antics, just as I had. The result was that I felt joy myself, especially knowing that my husband was having a good time. The last thing I wanted was for him to feel guilty about having fun with Cam.

Do not be reluctant to share your challenges and difficulties with the person in your care.

Every relationship is different, but sharing your struggles with the person you're caring for can make the two of you closer. Many caregivers are reluctant to share their difficulties for fear of making the person in their care feel worse. But sharing your struggles and even your sorrows can make your loved one feel as if he or she is giving you emotional support. As a result, not only will you get that support, but the person you're caring for will feel as if he or she is contributing to the well-being of the relationship.

Do not become isolated yourself, even if the person you care for is housebound.

Caregivers are often as isolated as the person in their care. If this is the case for you, consider asking someone to step in for part of a day so that you can get out in the world for a while. Many communities have respite programs that provide support for caregivers. In my town, there's an organization called Citizens Who Care that has a program called "Time Off for Caregivers." Volunteers come to people's houses for the specific purpose of giving caregivers the opportunity to go out and visit with other people or do something special for themselves.

There are also online support groups for caregivers that can help to ease your isolation. Connecting with others in this way benefits both you and the person you're caring for because it puts you in touch with others who understand the challenges you're facing. This can lift your spirits and renew your commitment; it can also provide valuable information that will make it easier for you to carry out your responsibilities.

Do not neglect your own health.

In chapter 25, I suggested that the person under your care be on the lookout for health problems that you might be developing, and which you might be ignoring due to your focus on him or her. Bottom line: you can't be an effective caregiver if you don't take care of yourself physically and emotionally. Ignoring your own health can negatively impact you and the person you're caring for. Caring attention to what's going on with you physically and mentally is essential to being a good caregiver for another. It's an act of compassion for both you and your loved one.

To find a measure of peace in your role as a caregiver, it helps to keep in mind that you cannot fix the person in your care. Doctors can't fix your loved one, so how can you be expected to? And you also can't keep your loved one from experiencing life's ups and downs, including sadness and sorrow.

I recommend that you come up with some equanimity phrases to remind you that, as much as you love the person in your care, you can't make his or her life conflict- and suffering-free. These are some of the phrases I use when I find myself embarking on the fruitless endeavor to try and fix the lives of my loved ones so that they'll never have to experience tough times. I hope some of the phrases resonate with you as a caregiver:

- ► I love you, but I cannot keep you from feeling disappointed and sad.
- ► I hope that along with your sorrows, you're able to experience joy.
- ► May you find peace and well-being in the midst of your difficult circumstances.

40

Lessons for the Healthy from the Land of the Sick

Everything has been figured out, except how to live.

—JEAN-PAUL SARTRE

PEOPLE WHO ARE in good health can learn a lot by paying attention to those who are chronically ill. I still hope to regain my health. Should that day come, the lessons I've learned in the land of the sick will accompany me to the land of the healthy.

Expanding your thinking beyond your personal problems helps you accept the life you have.

I used to think that I'd been singled out because of this illness, as if the world were being unfair to me personally. This gave rise to anger and resentment. Over the years, I've learned the value of going beyond this narrow self-focused thinking. I haven't been singled out; in every household on the planet, in every generation, in every era throughout history, people have experienced unexpected upheavals in their lives. Expanding my thinking in this way has helped me accept my life as it is.

If I recover my health, I'm determined to maintain this broader perspective. My life—just like everyone else's—will be a mixture of pleasant and unpleasant experiences, successes and disappointments, joys and sorrows.

Your identity need not be tied to a job title.

When illness forced me to spend my days in the bedroom instead of the classroom, I continued to think of myself as a law professor long after it was clear that this was no longer in the cards for me. I clung to that identity as if it were a life raft, repeating to myself over and over in a panic, "If I'm not a law professor, who am I?"

One day, out of a combination of frustration and exhaustion, I let go of the label "law professor" and the identity that went along with it. To my surprise and relief, I felt liberated, as if I'd put down a heavy load. This left me free to create a new life for myself. Now I look for fulfillment in a broader range of interests and activities, without the need to call myself something that's important-sounding.

Whether you're healthy or not, I hope you won't limit your identity to a job title. Doing so may keep you from exploring the abundance of life's possibilities and lead you to believe that your fulfillment is dependent on what you do for a living.

Dwelling on the past and worrying about the future are recipes for stress and anxiety.

I'm not suggesting that you can't learn from the past or that skillful planning for the future isn't worthwhile, but it's wise to be mindful that this type of thinking can become unproductive. For many years after becoming ill, I spent most of my days stuck in regret about a life I could no longer lead or lost in worry about a life I couldn't predict with any degree of certainty. I was miserable.

Then I remembered a book I'd read in the early 1990s: *Present Moment, Wonderful Moment* by Thich Nhat Hanh. In it, he wrote:

> When we settle into the present moment, we can see beauties and wonders right before our eyes—a newborn baby, the sun rising in the sky.

Encouraged by his words, I began to practice staying in the present moment. I devised an exercise I call "drop it." It's an alternative practice to the four-step approach I've discussed in previous chapters. If it suits you, use it! Here's how it works.

When you become aware that you're stuck in regret about the past, or that you're overcome with worry about what the future holds, gently but firmly say, "Drop it." Then immediately direct your attention to some current sensory input. It could be something you see or smell. It could be the physical sensation of your feet on the ground or of your breath coming in and out of your body. Dropping a stressful train of thought about the past or the future and relaxing into the present moment is a relief. And adding a slight smile can bring with it a sense of peace and well-being.

Note that there are two parts to this practice. First, saying "drop it," and then, turning your attention to a sensory experience in the present moment. It's important not to forget that second part. Without it, you're just barking a command at yourself; if you're like me, ordering yourself not to think or feel something makes those very thoughts or feelings stick like glue in your mind. That's why, after saying "drop it," it's important to turn your attention to something else in your field of awareness.

Those who are healthy can also benefit from "drop it" practice.

After all, no one is likely to make it through the day without his or her mind hosting a stressful thought or two about the past:

"I should have been more chatty at lunch instead of sitting there like a dunce."

"I shouldn't have stayed so long at my friend's house; I'm sure I wore out my welcome."

Notice how thoughts about the past often contain self-critical "shoulds" and "shouldn'ts." These serve only to make you feel inadequate, as if you're not living up to some ideal standard of behavior, but those standards tend to be unrealistically high. Who is ever 100 percent satisfied with everything he or she said at a social function? No one I've ever met. Who is able to perfectly calculate how long to stay at someone's house? No one. Dwelling on the past and adding a negative self-judgment into the mix only add stress and anxiety to life.

You're also unlikely to have made it this far in your day without your mind hosting a stressful thought or two about the future.

I faced this head-on in the fall of 2014 when I suddenly found myself waiting for the results of seven medical tests in a three-week period. Understandably, at times, I felt anxious and worried. I made matters worse, however, when I began spinning stressful stories about the future even though I could not possibly know what it had in store for me. It amazed me how this mental chatter ranged from the embarrassingly trivial (how will I keep up my Facebook posts if I have to be hospitalized?) to serious considerations (how will this impact my family?).

During those difficult weeks, I relied heavily on "drop it" practice and on tonglen. When I became aware that I was lost in worst-case scenarios about the future, I gently but firmly said, "drop it." Then I immediately turned my attention to something that was going on in the present moment. Sometimes I saw, as Thich Nhat Hanh said, beauties and wonders right before my eyes.

I also practiced tonglen (which is discussed in detail in earlier chapters) by breathing in the worry and anxiety of everyone everywhere who was waiting for test results and breathing out—to them and to myself—all the compassion and serenity I could summon up. This helped me feel connected to the millions of people who were in my same situation. This special bond helped me accept with equanimity that, although waiting for test results is definitely one of life's unpleasant experiences, it's one that almost everyone must endure at one time or another in life. The best we can do is try to keep our attention in the present moment and call on our storehouse of patience and compassion.

I'm grateful that I had "drop it" and tonglen as practices to help me through those challenging weeks. Maybe you're in good health and are waiting for the results of a different kind of test: an entry exam for a job, for example. You need not be chronically ill to benefit from practices that help stem worry and anxiety.

Taking "I," me," and "mine" out of your thinking can keep you from treating unpleasant physical and emotional states as permanent features of who you are.

In chapter 24, "The Uncertainty of It All," I wrote about the practice of reformulating your thoughts by taking out self-referential terms, such as "I," "me," and "mine." To do this, you treat how you're feeling at the moment as being the result of the temporary coming together of causes and conditions in your life, as opposed to being due to some permanent quality of yourself.

This perspective can benefit everyone, including those in good health. Here's an example of how I've used this practice.

Because I'm home almost all the time, often by myself, I decided in the spring of 2014 to bring new life into the house. We got a puppy and named her Scout. My husband drove to pick her up when she was twelve weeks old. Because the drive was too long for me, our friend Richard was kind enough to accompany him.

While they were on the road, I lay down for my nap. My plan was to be in as good shape as possible when Scout arrived. But I couldn't sleep. In fact, I couldn't even rest. Unexpectedly, I was overcome with anxiety about what was about to happen. "I can't believe how anxious I am," I thought. The anxiety then triggered an avalanche of stressful stories: "Will I be able to adequately exercise a puppy? Who will train her? How will I ensure a quiet environment for my nap and for sleep at night?"

As I lay there, it became clear that this so-called nap was making matters worse, because lying still in the quiet had become fertile ground for generating these stressful stories. After about a half hour, I decided to try the practice of taking self-referential terms out of my thinking. (Note that all of the stressful thoughts contained the word "I" in them!) And so instead of thinking "I can't believe how anxious I am," I changed it to "Anxiety is happening" and "Anxiety is present." Then I took a moment to explore how anxiety felt—in both my body and my mind.

First, I noticed that my body was tense and that the muscles in my neck were particularly tight. Then I reflected on how several causes and conditions had come together at this moment in time to create the anxiety I was experiencing: the uncertainty of the demands that a new puppy would bring; the unpredictability of my illness from day-to-day; the fact that this was the very day my husband was picking her up; my determination that this nap would put me in good shape to greet her. As I reflected on this, I kept repeating "Anxiety is happening" and "Anxiety is present." There was no need to identify with this anxiety as an intrinsic quality of who I was. It just happened to be what was going on at the moment.

The result of reformulating my thinking in this way was that the anxiety lost its oppressive feel and the tension in my body relaxed. A feeling of spaciousness arose in which the anxiety was nothing more than a fluid emotional state—coming and going, arising and passing—as opposed to being a permanent feature of this person Toni Bernhard. I thought, "Yes, anxiety is present; that's okay. Just let it be." As I lay on my bed, the anxiety eventually gave way to a pleasant feeling of curiosity; instead of feeling anxious, I was suddenly interested in seeing how life with Scout would unfold.

This perspective—that what happens in life is the result of causes and conditions that are ever-changing, out of your control, and need not be taken personally—is helpful in a broad range of settings. It was another practice I relied on during the three weeks I spent waiting for test results. When worry and anxiety arose, I worked on describing them without the use of self-referential terms. And so I'd say "Worry is happening" or "Anxiety is present." Doing this kept me from identifying with what I was feeling, and that made it easier for the worry and anxiety to lift and blow away—over and over again.

Whether you're chronically ill or not, I hope you'll try this practice. It can help you "go with the flow," instead of treating an unpleasant physical or emotional state as a permanent feature of who you are.

Less is more.

Before I got sick, I was an accumulator. My life was filled with *stuff*: unopened books and magazines that sat unread; CDs; jewelry; knickknacks and trinkets; clothing and all its accessories (shoes, belts, scarves). Since becoming sick, I've learned that less is more. As a result, if someone admires something, unless it's a special item that I'm saving for my children or grandchildren, I give it away. So be careful if you come to my house; if you say you like something, odds are, it's about to be yours.

I love to give things away. I have less but I feel as if I have more, because I have the satisfaction of knowing that I've made someone happy and that something that was once mine will now be put to better use. If I woke up tomorrow morning with my health restored, I wouldn't change this behavior. It carries with it a newfound sense of freedom.

Clean is better than neat.

My house isn't neat, but it's relatively clean. The limitations imposed by my illness have forced me to choose between the two because I can't manage both; I can have neat, or I can have clean. I've chosen clean. This means that if I wipe down a refrigerator shelf, I feel good about it, even though I know its contents will still be in disarray when I'm done. When I do laundry, if I've managed to get the sheets and some detergent into the washer, I consider it a job well done even if the sheets emerge from the dryer only to be casually shoved onto a shelf (clean but not neat!) until I need them.

Rushing to judgment about others can lead to painful misunderstandings.

When I got sick, I rushed to judgment about friends who didn't keep in touch. I assumed they no longer cared about me. As I've written about in earlier chapters, most of my assumptions were way off base. I could have saved myself a lot of suffering if I'd kept that Don't-Know Mind I wrote about in chapter 21. As Korean Zen teacher Seung Sahn said, "If you keep a don't-know mind, then your mind is clear like space and clear like a mirror."

Whether in good health or not, we're all experts at clouding our minds with stressful stories about other people—stories in which we impute motives and intentions that more often than not have no basis in fact. In truth, we don't know what's happening in another person's life unless we inquire about it. Yes, it may be time to let a relationship go and move on, but before doing so, consider asking yourself whether you've rushed to judgment without checking out what might really be going on.

Paying attention to your body's needs is of utmost importance.

Before I got sick, I lived mostly in my mind. I thought of my body and mind as separate and disconnected. Like most people, I'd been taught "mind over matter," as if the body were a slave to the mind, carrying out its directives. As a result of that belief, I ignored my body when it sent me signals that would have been beneficial to me, such as to slow down or to get more sleep. Being chronically ill has made me more conscious of the interconnectedness of mind and body. I can feel, for example, how emotions are felt in the body and how mental stress can exacerbate physical symptoms.

Should I regain my health, I'll stay embodied—I'll stay *in body*. I'll listen to what it's saying to me, and I'll remember to appreciate what an extraordinary organism it is. Even when I'm struggling mightily with this illness, my heart keeps beating, my blood keeps circulating, my lungs keep taking in oxygen.

The body may be the most wondrous instrument in the world, but it's also fragile.

When I saw people on television stranded in the heat and humidity on the cement freeway overpasses in New Orleans after the levees broke, I thought, "I would not survive in that situation." When I see pictures of Sudanese refugees walking days on end to find food and water, I think, "They would have had to leave me behind."

It's a sobering thought and not, I believe, one that people who are healthy realize is the case.

Illness is the great equalizer.

My health care provider serves the indigent in several counties. When I have an appointment, I share the waiting room with the homeless and the affluent. People graciously give up their chairs to others in need. People admire each other's children. They engage in friendly small talk. We know we're in this together.

When you're chronically ill, barriers fall. Illness and pain don't care about your background or your life circumstances: whether you're financially secure or struggling to pay the rent, whether you have an advanced degree or a high school diploma, whether you have plenty of support from others or are utterly alone. Should I regain my health, I'll never lose sight of the fact that, underneath the trappings of society and our particular life circumstances, we're all equals on the path of life.

Being kind to yourself is the best medicine.

As I've written about several times in this book, when I first became chronically ill, I was not kind to myself. I thought my body had betrayed me. I thought my mind was weak because I couldn't will myself back to health. My inner critic was in full voice. It took several years, but I finally learned to treat myself with kindness and compassion.

Once I began speaking to myself in a caring voice, I realized how much I could have benefitted from this supportive self-talk *before* I got sick. In my early years of teaching, I felt inadequate in the classroom. I judged myself harshly even though I worked as hard as I could to be a good professor. I wish I'd known to say to myself something like "Such a dedicated teacher, working so hard to do the best for my students."

Healthy or not, no one's life is without bumps in the road. When the going gets rough, instead of blaming yourself for your difficulties, try to see them as an inevitable part of the human experience. Then take a big dose of that best of medicines: self-compassion. It will heal your mind and bring you a measure of peace no matter what your circumstances.

Cosmically, there's no difference between weekdays and weekends, or between regular days and holidays.

It's just sunrise, sunset, sunrise, sunset. Treasure and enjoy.

VIII. Last But Not Least

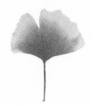

41

True Confessions

Waking up to who you are requires letting go of
who you imagine yourself to be.

—ALAN WATTS

WHETHER HEALTHY OR not, all of us face the challenge at some point in our lives of letting go of who we imagine ourselves to be. With chronic illness, however, that challenge may be thrust upon us before we're prepared for it—indeed before we even see it coming. Waking up to who we are requires honesty and courage. Although these confessions—some lighthearted, some not—are personal, I offer them on behalf of everyone who is chronically ill.

When I have a medical problem not related to my chronic illness, I'm likely to hide it from others.

In chapter 7, "Dealing with Tough Choice after Tough Choice," I raised the ongoing challenge of deciding how much to share with family and friends about our chronic conditions. We may badly be in need of their support, but at the same time we don't want our medical struggles to negatively impact our relationships.

So what happens when we develop a health issue that's not related to our chronic illness? When this happens to me, I confess that, whenever possible, I keep quiet about it. The reason is simple: I'm concerned that the people I care about the most will roll their eyes and silently think, "*Another* medical problem?"

I'm aware that this is probably not an accurate assessment of how my family and friends would react. Even so, because it took some of them a while to accept that I'm sick all the time, I don't want to spring on them that I now have an unrelated issue with my health. So I leave well enough alone, but I also confess that keeping things private in this way increases my sense of isolation.

Sometimes I envy those who are more seriously ill than I am.

I know a woman who has a progressive disease that keeps her confined to a wheelchair and affects her ability to speak clearly. And yet she and her husband are able to travel. They visit their children who live out of town, and they go on vacations. In her immobility, in some ways, she's more mobile than I am; her symptoms don't keep her confined to the bed or the house. I've sometimes envied her even though it's likely that I'll outlive her. It's hard to admit to this feeling but, after all, I am confessing.

I love my bed.

I know it's better not to stay in bed or even on the bed if I don't need to, but I confess: I love my bed. Aside from its traditional uses, I never realized what a multifunctional, versatile piece of furniture it is.

My bed makes a great office; it's where I do all my writing.

There's plenty of space to spread out books and notes, and a laptop fits nicely on my reclined body. In addition, none of the many expensive ergonomically designed office chairs that were provided for me at my other places of work came close to being as comfortable as the combination of my soft mattress and my customized, self-arranged, multi-pillow set-up.

My bed is also my entertainment and my craft center. I can watch television, including movies and shows on DVD and streamed from Netflix. (And my multi-pillow arrangement is more comfortable than any theater seat I can remember, not to mention that I can take a bathroom break anytime without missing a thing.) I can listen to music and to audiobooks. I can play Scrabble on my computer. I can crochet. So many possibilities!

And my bed makes a great dog playground: tug-of-war, tickle the tummy. My favorite game is something I call "bed rats" (I don't know where the name comes from). I jerk my hand around under the quilt and grab at my dog's paws and legs. She gets crazy happy—barking and wagging her tail, while playfully biting at a hand she can't see. It's not so good for the quilt, but it's a cheap quilt.

Finally, my bed also serves as the perfect intermediate stopping place for dishes that are on their way from my lap to the kitchen. Cautionary note: bed as dish depository and bed as dog playground should not be attempted simultaneously.

I've become an expert eavesdropper.

I'm rarely able to hang out in the living room for the entire time that family or friends are visiting. When I retreat to my bedroom, instead of listening to an audiobook or turning on the television, I eavesdrop on the conversation going on in the living room. I've even been known to lie down on the rug right inside the bedroom door so as to be able to hear more clearly. Sometimes people are even talking about me—what a bonus! I'm not proud of this new skill as an eavesdropper, but it reflects how hard it is to leave the company of others when I'm having a good time.

I worry that I'm no longer competent out in the world.

Sometimes I don't know what's appropriate to wear. I have a night-shirt that, to me, looks nice enough to wear in public. The problem is, it almost goes down to my knees, and so I'm concerned that, to others, it looks like the nightshirt that it really is. A few years ago, I bought some footwear online from L.L.Bean called "scuffs." They sure looked like shoes to me, but the first time I wore them out, someone diplomatically pointed out that I'd left the house in slip-pers. I'm left wondering two things: just what *are* "scuffs"? And, in my isolation, has a whole new language for clothing passed me by?

If I have to drive somewhere, I try to make sure I won't have to fill up on gas. I don't understand the new procedure, even though my husband has demonstrated it to me several times. The problem is, there's always such a long interval between when he last showed me and when I'm the one who needs to put gas in the car that I forget his instructions: Do I swipe my credit card before or after I put the gas in? Which way do I hold the card so as to get a proper swipe? How do I get the nozzle to stay in the tank without holding on to it? How do I take it out without spilling gas all over the side of the car? I'm clueless.

Then there was the time I took my friend Kari to an early dinner as a thank-you for editing the manuscript for my book *How to Wake Up*. The bill came, and I took it out of the folder. Looking it over, I was puzzled. I said to Kari, "I don't see a place to add in a tip." She politely pointed out that I was supposed to put my credit card in the folder and that, after the server swiped the card, I'd get a new bill with space for a tip. Wow. I used to know that. On a bad day, this worry can escalate into fear that I'll be treated like a child if I'm not right on top of an interaction.

I don't know what groceries cost.

I'm fortunate that my husband does our grocery shopping. The problem is, he's been doing it for so many years that I've lost track of what things cost. Sometimes he playfully names an item and asks me what I think he paid for it: a quart of milk, a bunch of bananas, toilet paper. I was consistently far off the mark until I figured out a way to beat his game. I make a silent guess at what I think the item would cost, and then multiply the number by four. That almost always gets me close.

I'm content to be a walking contradiction.

Walt Whitman famously said, "Do I contradict myself? Very well, then I contradict myself, I am large, I contain multitudes." Contradictory feelings are normal. On a retreat many years ago, Buddhist teacher Jack Kornfield referred to life as "happy-sad." Those words resonated strongly with me. I can be happy and sad at the same time. For example, I'm sad that I'm sick, but I'm happy that I'm able to connect with others online who understand what this life is like.

And I can be disappointed and, at the same time, feel okay about my life. In 2012, I was too sick to attend the thirtieth reunion of my law school class, even though it took place in the town where I live. I badly wanted to go, so I was disappointed that I had to miss it. And yet, at the same time, I felt okay about it. Yes, being sick is unpleasant, but I have a decent place to live, a caring partner, and a sweet little dog to keep me company when there's no human around. So life is okay.

Making room in my heart for contradictory feelings is an equanimity practice; I feel more at peace when I let them live side-by-side in harmony.

At times I'd like to trade some of my functionality for a disability that's visible to others.

It's hard to confess to this desired trade-off: less functionality in exchange for not having to respond to "But you don't *look* sick." But there you have it.

Sometimes I park in a disabled spot as a favor to the nondisabled.

I have a disabled parking placard. Because I'm able to walk short distances, unless I'm having a particularly bad day, I don't park in a disabled space. That said, there's one parking lot in town where it's usually impossible to find a place to park *unless* you have that placard. Then I use a disabled space to leave one of the few "regular" spots for the nondisabled—which always makes me feel guilty and altruistic at the same time.

I listen to audiobooks the way people listen to music they love: over and over and over.

I'm always being told that I simply must read this new book or that new book. I nod as if I'll keep it in mind. What I don't share is that I'm busy listening to *A Room with a View* for the tenth time, or to an Alexander McCall Smith book for the umpteenth time, or to a P. D. James mystery again even though I know whodunit.

These aren't necessarily great novels. They're just books in which I've made friends with the characters. I'm pretty isolated, but these are people I *can* hang out with. I'd like to help Miss Lucy Honeychurch out when she's in yet another one of her muddles. I'd like to be on detective Adam Dalgliesh's crime-solving team.

And I'd love to be in Botswana, sharing bush tea with McCall Smith's No. 1 ladies' detective, Mma Ramotswe. I have the same relationship to a few movies. *Gosford Park* comes to mind. I want Maggie Smith to come over and insult *me* with her acerbic wit. For the privilege, I'll even play the role of her lady's maid and dutifully put sliced cucumbers on her eyelids.

I may have an unhealthy dependence on the internet... and I don't care.

When my internet connection goes down, I'm immediately on edge. Then a light bulb goes on in my brain and I think, "No problem. I'll just Google 'troubleshooting your internet connection.'" Then I realize I can't Google anything. Next, I think, "Well, at least I can email a friend in town and see if her internet is down too." Then I realize I can't email anybody.

The last time this happened, with a sigh, I said to myself, "I'll treat this as an equanimity practice and calmly let things be until the internet comes back up. Meanwhile, I'll relax by finishing that British TV drama I've been streaming on Netflix." I turned on the television and tried to access Netflix. Nope. Turns out, Netflix only streams when my internet is working.

These efforts on my part lead me to conclude that I may have an unhealthy dependence on the internet. This reflection is a brief one, however, as it is immediately followed by the thought, "I don't care. Just get my internet up and running, whoever or whatever you are that's keeping it from working. And I mean NOW!"

I don't shower every day.

This would have been unimaginable to me before I got sick. But you know what? My skin seems to appreciate it.

Dresser drawers are my chosen solution for decluttering my living space.

Do you want less clutter but are too sick or in too much pain to wrap your mind around all those YouTube videos on how to declutter your living space? When deciding what to do with an item, we're supposed to carefully consider three alternatives: give it away, throw it away, or keep it. And if we decide to keep it, we're supposed to find its one and only proper place. Well, there's a fourth alternative: shove it! Yes, out of sight in a drawer *is* out of mind.

I cut my own hair.

No, I don't know what I'm doing, although I did find a YouTube video on cutting bangs that helped. It also helps that my hair is wavy, so mistakes don't show unless they're egregious. I don't do it to save money. I started doing it because it was more taxing for me to listen to the real-life dramas of the hairstylist I was going to than it was to sit on a chair in front of a mirror and spend forty-five minutes hacking away. Funny thing is, I receive the occasional compliment on my haircut!

When I'm alone, my eating habits are fit only for my dog to see.

I'm not sure I want everyone to know this but, when I'm alone, I lick the bowls and plates after I've eaten from them. After all, there's food to be had there, and every dish licked is a dish that's easier to wash.

Even when I really want to see people, I'm relieved when they have to cancel.

The reason is simple: their cancellation also cancels the payback I'll have to go through as a result of the visit. Because there's not a day when I'm not sick or in pain, sometimes I'm willing to pay the price that a visit will cost so that I can spend some time with other people. Nonetheless, there's always a sense of relief when they cancel because then I know I've saved my body from payback.

In the fall of 2013, I committed to a few nearby events so that I could give a short talk on *How to Wake Up* when it was published. One afternoon, as I was getting dressed to go to an event at my local bookstore, I found myself saying to my body, "I'm sorry for forcing you to do this." I was taken aback by these words until I realized that, although I'd freely chosen to do this event, if the bookstore had called and cancelled, I confess I'd have been relieved.

The author of *How to Be Sick* doesn't always know how to be sick.

In January of 2012, I found myself going rapidly downhill. I was waking up feeling more sick than usual, and all day long had intense symptoms. I thought about whether I'd made any changes in my life that might have triggered this downward spiral: a new medication, a change in diet. I couldn't come up with anything, and so I began to get scared that my "baseline" had gone down a notch or two.

I tried to hide what was happening from my husband because I didn't want him to worry. One evening, I could tell that he knew what was going on. I began sobbing and shared with him my frustration and my fears. As we talked, I realized that my worsened condition had nothing to do with any external changes in my life. I had simply stopped taking good care of myself. When getting up in the morning, instead of asking "How can I take care of myself today?" I was asking "How can I push my limits today?" As a result, I was overextending myself in every way: visiting with people for too long, pushing against my naptime and my bedtime, staying on the computer for too long.

I'd forgotten to follow my own advice on "how to be sick."

Within days of beginning to take care of myself again, I'd returned to my baseline.

If you're like me, some days, you're just plain weary of being chronically ill. I remember seeing my primary care doctor a few years ago for my usual three-month follow-up (fourteen years of "follow-ups"—there's dark humor to *that* notion!). As usual, he asked how I was doing. I slowly shook my head and said, "I'm sick of being sick." I half expected him to say, "What? The author of *How to Be Sick* is sick of being sick?" But he didn't. He understood.

The poet Carl Sandburg wrote, "Life is like an onion; you peel it off one layer at a time, and sometimes you weep." Writing this chapter was like peeling an onion for me. A few of my confessions brought tears to my eyes. I decided to treat them as cleansing tears: this is how my life is, so I might as well face up to it by peeling off the layers and seeing what's going on. I feel certain that those of you who are chronically ill share most of my confessions. My only regret is that I can't hear yours.

42

My Heartfelt Wishes for the Chronically Ill

If we cannot change the way we are, the skill of life becomes learning how to feel deep love and care for what is flowing through our fingers, even while letting it go.

—ANDREW OLENDZKI

OF COURSE, my first wish for those of you who are chronically ill is for your health to be restored. For some, this is a realistic possibility; for others, only a distant dream. It's a challenge to mindfully walk that middle path between being proactive about your health—always trying to improve it—but at the same time, accepting the way you are so that you can make the best of each day.

And so, although *restored health* is my number one wish, here are my other wishes for the chronically ill.

May you accept with equanimity whatever support your family and friends are able to offer.

When I share with family and friends what it's like to live with chronic illness, I don't care if they use the perfect words in response. I just hope for something like "I'm so sorry" or "It must be hard." Then I know I've been heard and believed, and that goes a long way toward making me feel okay about the course my life has taken.

My wish is that you'll be at peace with whatever support those you feel closest to are able to offer. This includes the possibility that some of them may never educate themselves about what you're going through; I've had this happen and, at first, it hurt badly every time. It took me a while to realize that other people's unwillingness or inability to understand my life is about them, not about me. I hope that if there are people in your life who don't make the effort you wish they would to understand what you're going through, you won't blame yourself.

A theme that has run throughout this book is that we can't force other people to behave the way we want them to. Even though it may hurt when we feel let down by others, it helps to recognize that the suffering we're experiencing is coming from our own wanting minds. It helps because that wanting is something we can work on overcoming.

In the end, all we can do is put forth our best effort to educate family and friends about what life is like for us, and then, with equanimity, either let them slip out of our lives without bitterness or, if that's not possible, work on being content with what they're able to offer.

May you find a doctor who treats you as a partner in your health care.

I hope you have a doctor who isn't intimidated if you know more about your illness than he or she does. In this internet age, it's not unusual for people who are chronically ill to become experts on their own conditions. I'm fortunate that my primary care doctor welcomes learning from me and is open to trying treatments that I suggest. In addition, when I have an appointment with another physician, my primary doctor helps me figure out how to explain my illness in a way that maximizes the chances that I'll get the best care possible. I feel as if we're in this together.

I hope you're able to find a doctor who will work with you as a partner in your health care.

May you treat yourself with compassion over this unexpected turn your life has taken.

Chronic pain and illness can turn your life upside down. When this happens, it's essential to your peace of mind and sense of well-being to avoid getting trapped by self-blame. The best way to do this is to wrap yourself in a protective cloak of compassion.

I include many self-compassion exercises in my books because they're my personal go-to practices when I'm having trouble coping with being chronically ill, especially when the thought arises that maybe it's my fault that I'm sick. That thought—or any negative self-judgment—is a signal to work on making my loyalty to myself unconditional.

One of the most effective ways to do this is to speak silently to myself, using whatever compassionate words fit the moment: "It's hard to be in pain and not have an easy 'fix' available"; "I'm doing the best I can to cope with feeling sick all the time"; "My sweet body, working so hard to support me." As I say these words, I often stroke my arm or my cheek. It never fails to ease my emotional pain.

No matter how difficult a day you're having, may you keep
your heart open for a ray of sunshine.

That ray can take many forms: the sight of a beautiful print on the
wall, the sound of a child's laughter, the sensation of warm water
on your skin. I like to look at my dog for that ray of sunshine. I
see her and say to myself, "She doesn't know I'm sick." For some
reason, knowing that she thinks I'm perfectly fine makes me feel a
bit better, no matter how tough a day I'm having. It also inspires
me to look around to see what the world might have to offer this
"perfectly fine" person. In the words of Joseph Campbell:

> We must let go of the life we have planned, so as to accept
> the one that is waiting for us.

Some days, all that's waiting for me is a funny movie on TV to
distract me from my symptoms, but that's okay. A good distraction
can serve as that ray of sunshine—and a distraction always feels
better than clinging to the life we planned but can no longer lead.

May you make peace with the possibility that you'll be
chronically ill for the rest of your life.

One day in 2013, I had a moment of truth: I realized that I might
be chronically ill for the rest of my life. I've tried dozens of treatments; none of them has cleared up the flu-like symptoms that I
live with day in and day out. When the thought arose "I might feel
like this for the rest of my life," surprisingly, instead of feeling sad
and depressed, I felt liberated, as if a great burden had lifted: the
burden to get better.

Without that burden, I felt free to get on with the life I have
instead of fighting a constant and exhausting battle for what, in the
end, I may not be able to get—my health restored. Don't get me
wrong: I'm still actively looking for new treatments, but I'm also

newly open to the possibility that there might not be a treatment out there that's going to work for me. This openness is helping me be at peace with my life as it is.

In the middle 1990s, I listened to a talk on cassette tape given by Pema Chödrön. She was discussing a slogan from a Tibetan Buddhist teaching called the Seven Points of Mind Training: "Give up all hope of fruition." I had my own interpretation of what it might mean: "Give up striving for enlightenment" or something along those lines. But here's how Pema Chödrön interpreted it. Very simply, she said:

- Give up all hope of fruition.
- Give up all hope.
- Give up.
- Give.

I never forgot these words even though I never quite understood them. I can see why some readers may balk at the idea "Give up all hope" and even more at the idea "Give up." Yet during that moment in 2013, I felt as if I finally understood what Pema Chödrön was getting at: even as we continue to look for ways to improve our health, the only path to peace is to give up the painful, impulsive striving to reach that goal.

Finally, there's that simple word "Give" at the end of her commentary. To me, it means giving myself to the life I have as opposed to tying my happiness to a goal that might not be attainable. It also means giving to others; when I do that, even though I'm chronically ill, my life has purpose.

May you look upon your life as an adventure, despite your illness and pain.

In chapter 40, I wrote about getting a puppy. I wanted to do something adventurous with my life since I'm home almost all the time.

Two months after Scout arrived, she broke her right front leg in two different places. The repair required separate surgeries on successive days. Scout was in the hospital for five days and then needed extensive physical rehabilitation.

Even before the surgeries were performed, I started worrying about whether I'd be able to take care of her after she came home. Given my illness, could I adequately care for a puppy who'd have to be strictly confined for at least two months? Could I keep her from re-injuring her leg? If I were home alone, how would I get her to the vet in an emergency? Bringing a puppy into my life was suddenly feeling like a disaster.

As I lay on my bed, spinning these stressful stories, this thought popped into my mind: "I wanted to embark on an adventure to shake up my life. *Scout is my adventure.*" This simple thought changed my perspective about what lay ahead. I began to look upon the weeks to come as part of the adventure of having brought a puppy into my life. Instead of worrying, I began to plan for her homecoming. Where was the best place to keep her confined? What could I buy or borrow that would make the experience easier?

Not surprisingly, taking care of Scout was tough at times, especially given my own poor health. And yet the difficulties that arose weren't the ones I'd been anticipating. All that fretting about the future served only to make an unpleasant experience worse for me.

Inspired by this experience, I decided to try treating my life as an adventure, even on days when I feel so sick that it's clearly not the adventure I'd have signed up for. Being chronically ill has been one of the biggest challenges of my life. I hope one day to look back on it as also one of my biggest adventures. I wish the same for you.

May you not mind what happens.

This oddly worded wish comes from a story about the philosopher and spiritual teacher Jiddu Krishnamurti. In the middle of a talk he was giving in Ojai, California, he suddenly paused, leaned forward and whispered to those in attendance: "Do you want to know what my secret is? *I don't mind what happens.*"

It's a tall order to not mind what happens. Some days, I mind so much that I happened to get sick that I can't see past the overwhelming desire to have my health restored. Yet even in the midst of this painful desire, I know that, for me, the path to peace and contentment is to not mind that chronic illness has happened in my life.

And so whenever this intense desire to be healthy takes hold, I gently acknowledge its presence, and then I imagine how I'd feel if I didn't mind what happens. Sometimes this imagining is enough to break the spell of the desire to have my health restored. And when I can truly rest in that place of not minding what happens—even if it's only for a moment—I feel free.

May you "make the best use of what is in your power and take the rest as it happens."

This phrase comes from Epictetus, who was born a slave in 55 AD in what is modern-day Turkey. As a young man, he gained his freedom, moved to Rome, and began to teach philosophy. When philosophers were banished from Rome in 89 AD, he left and started his own school in northwest Greece, where he lived and taught for the rest of his life.

Despite seemingly insurmountable hardships, Epictetus lived a life of purpose, dedicated to helping others. My heartfelt wish is that all of you learn to "make the best use of what is in your power and take the rest as it happens." The way I see it, there's no higher purpose in life than to use what's in our power to be kind and helpful to ourselves and others, and to be at peace with taking the rest as it happens.

Afterword

Dear Readers,

I wrote in chapter 23 that my husband and I don't have the questionable luxury of dealing with variety in my health issues. Now we do. As I was completing the final editing of this book, I was diagnosed with breast cancer. Since then, I've been undergoing treatment and the prognosis is good. When I was first diagnosed, I was angry that this happened on top of my chronic illness. "If only I weren't already sick, I'd be able to handle this better," I protested.

The very opposite turned out to be true. The work I've done to find a measure of peace in the midst of chronic illness has been healing medicine for my heart and mind in this latest upside down turning of my life. For the first time, I've felt grateful that I got sick in 2001 because it prepared me for cancer with the caring attention that mindfulness asks of us, with compassion for myself and others who are living every day with uncertainty about what's going on in our bodies, and with equanimity in the face of wishing things were otherwise.

At times, I've been worried and scared, and some of the medical procedures and treatments have left me feeling sick, weak, and in pain. Even so, not far beneath the mental and physical suffering, there's a place of calm acceptance where, for the most part, I've felt at peace with this unexpected adventure that life had in store for me.

May we all find the place of peace within the turbulence of life.

With warmest wishes,

Toni

Acknowledgments

With appreciation and affection to the following:

Tim McNeill, Josh Bartok, Tony Lulek, Lydia Anderson, and everyone at Wisdom Publications, for their help and support. I'm grateful to Wisdom for publishing all three of my books.

Laura Cunningham of Wisdom, who worked with me on the final proofs for my first two books and then became my editor for this one. She was a joy to work with in every way. Laura can turn a mundane sentence into an elegant one, and she has the uncanny ability to edit a phrase so that it conveys the meaning I intended better than I was able to.

Lybi Ma, deputy editor, and the other editors at *Psychology Today* online, for their kindness in hosting my writing since April, 2011. Earlier versions of many chapters in this book initially appeared in my blog at *Psychology Today*.

My friends Kari Peterson and Elizabeth Zimmer, who, as they did with *How to Wake Up*, gave me invaluable feedback on the manuscript.

The many people, anonymous and not, who shared their stories with me and, by doing so, enriched the content of this book.

Dr. Paul Riggle, primary care doctor extraordinaire, for his continuing care and compassion.

Doctors Richard Bold, Megan Daly, and Barbara Galligan of the University of California–Davis Comprehensive Cancer Center. I could not be getting better care.

Nhi Nguyen and Greg Off, for their courage.

Dawn Daro, for her good company, year after year.

Sylvia Boorstein, for always making life sweeter.

Jazmín Ramos of Navidad, Jalisco, our unexpected housemate during her senior year at U.C. Davis, while I was not only working hard to prepare this book for publication but, out of the blue, was diagnosed with breast cancer. Her young spirit, her thoughtfulness, and her good company brightened my days at a time when I really needed it. Gracias desde lo más profundo de mi corazón, Jazmín.

Bridgett Bernhard and Brad Tyler, for being the spouses parents dream of for their children.

My granddaughters Malia and Cam, who don't want to change a thing about me and who ask the best questions.

Richard Farrell, for always being there for me.

And, as is true with my other books, this one would not exist without the help and support of my husband Tony—the love of my life and my best friend. *Tony, you are my heart's delight.*

About the Author

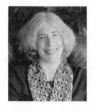 Toni Bernhard is the author of the award-winning *How to Be Sick: A Buddhist-Inspired Guide for the Chronically Ill and Their Caregivers* and *How to Wake Up: A Buddhist-Inspired Guide to Navigating Joy and Sorrow*. She's been interviewed on radio and for podcasts across the country and internationally. Her blog, "Turning Straw Into Gold," is hosted by *Psychology Today* online. She maintains a personal relationship with her many thousands of fans on Facebook and other social media sites.

Toni fell ill on a trip to Paris in 2001 with what doctors initially diagnosed as an acute viral infection. She has not recovered. Until forced by illness to retire, she was a law professor at the University of California–Davis, serving six years as the dean of students.

She has been a practicing Buddhist since the early 1990s. She lives in Davis with her husband, Tony, and their gray lab, Scout. Toni can be found online at tonibernhard.com.

Also Available by Toni Bernhard from Wisdom Publications

How to Be Sick
A Buddhist-Inspired Guide for the Chronically Ill and Their Caregivers
Foreword by Sylvia Boorstein

"Full of hopefulness and promise... this book is a perfect blend of inspiration and encouragement. Toni's engaging teaching style shares traditional Buddhist wisdom in a format that is accessible to all."
—*The Huffington Post*

How to Wake Up
A Buddhist-Inspired Guide to Navigating Joy and Sorrow

"This is a book for everyone."
—Alida Brill, author of *Dancing at the River's Edge*

About Wisdom Publications

WISDOM PUBLICATIONS is the leading publisher of classic and contemporary Buddhist books and practical works on mindfulness. Publishing books from all major Buddhist traditions, Wisdom is a nonprofit charitable organization dedicated to cultivating Buddhist voices the world over, advancing critical scholarship, and preserving and sharing Buddhist literary culture.

To learn more about us or to explore our other books, please visit our website at wisdompubs.org. You can subscribe to our eNewsletter, request a print catalog, and find out how you can help support Wisdom's mission either online or by writing to:

Wisdom Publications
199 Elm Street
Somerville, Massachusetts 02144 USA

You can also contact us at 617-776-7416 or info@wisdompubs.org.

Wisdom is a 501(c)(3) organization, and donations in support of our mission are tax deductible.

Wisdom Publications is affiliated with the Foundation for the Preservation of the Mahayana Tradition (FPMT).